Fit for Fatherhood

**Featuring
The Adrenaline Factor
Program**

Scott Macdonald

Published in Canada, May 2017 by The Art of Recovery

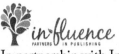

In partnership with Influence Publishing Inc.
ISBN: 9780995883000

Copyright © 2017 by Scott Macdonald
All rights reserved. No part of this publication may be reproduced, stored in or introduced into a retrieval system, or transmitted, in any form, or by any means (electronic, mechanical, photocopying, recording or otherwise) without the prior written permission of the publisher. This book is sold subject to the condition that it shall not, by way of trade or otherwise, be lent, resold, hired out, or otherwise circulated without the publisher's prior consent in any form of binding or cover other than that in which it is published and without a similar condition including this condition being imposed on the subsequent purchaser.

Book Cover Design: Scott Macdonald
Editor: Nina Shoroplova
Typeset: Greg Salisbury
Exercise Photographer: Rommel Ramirez

DISCLAIMER: This book has been created to inform individuals with an interest in taking back control of their own health and exercises. It is not intended in any way to replace other professional health care, but to support it. Readers of this publication agree that neither Scott Macdonald nor his publisher will be held responsible or liable for damages that may be alleged or resulting, directly, or indirectly, from their use of this publication. All external links are provided as a resource only and are not guaranteed to remain active for any length of time. Neither the publisher nor the author can be held accountable for the information provided by, or actions resulting from accessing these resources.

This book is dedicated to Shereesse who never gave up on me. It was your light I saw in the darkness and your love that pulled me from it.

Testimonial

"Tremendous! Acknowledging what every expectant father feels, but never admits. His Adrenaline Action Plan informs and inspires men to get in front of their fatherhood fears with leadership and participation. Wish I'd read this 35 years ago before my first son was born!"

Bob Mueller
Speaker, Best Selling Author, Emmy Award Winning Artist

Acknowledgements

I would like to thank Nina Shoroplova, my editor. I am appreciative for the respect and care you showed the work I have put into these pages.

I thank Lucinda Atwood for sharing her expertise and wisdom. Your support came at an important time to help finish this book.

I thank my wife Shereesse and our children Tara, Kyle, Logan, and Rourke for walking with me while I found my footing.

I thank my best friend Billy and his wife (my friend) Gertrude for bringing light and love to my life. Knowing you are in my life is a constant source of strength.

I thank my grandfather James who "won the war singlehandedly." You have taught me a special kind of patience and understanding.

Finally, I would like to thank my father, for everything. I love you, Dad.

Contents

Dedication III
Testimonial V
Acknowledgements VII

Chapter 1: Adjusting Your Perception 1

First Trimester 11
Chapter 2: Adrenalize Your Eating 11
Chapter 3: The Phase 1 Workout 21
Chapter 4: Supporting Your Partner in the First Trimester 41

Second Trimester 57
Chapter 5: The Three Main Food Categories 57
Chapter 6: The Phase 2 Workout 77
Chapter 7: Supporting Your Partner in the Second Trimester ... 87

Third Trimester 99
Chapter 8: Eating Well—7 Rules for Success 99
Chapter 9: The Phase 3 Workout 117
Chapter 10: Supporting Your Partner in the Third Trimester ... 129

Epilogue 137

Appendix A Exercise Details 139
Appendix B Stretch Details 183
Author Biography 189
About Scott 190

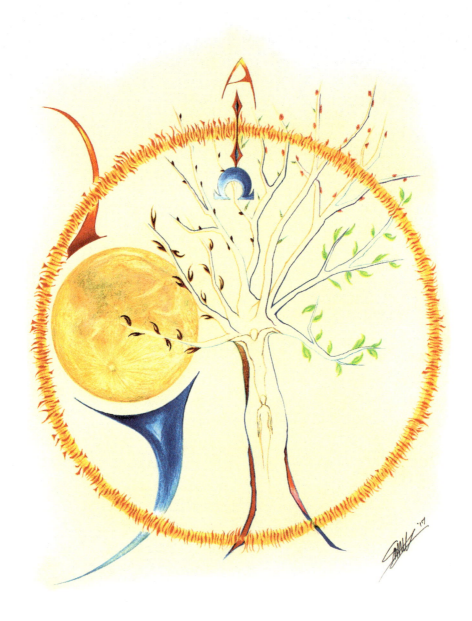

Chapter 1 Adjusting Your Perception

Congratulations! Whether planned or surprised, you are going to have a baby. You may be excited or terrified though probably both, but believe it or not your life has just taken a turn for the better.

    Congratulations also on picking up this book. Willingness to learn takes great strength and is a wonderful attribute to pass on to your child. This is a first step and the opportunity to make simple, powerful changes in your life. I invite you to continue with the strength, openness, and willingness you have shown this far and continue to apply it in reading this book. This book has been written to enhance your self-awareness. Further down in "The Roots of This Book," I have put some of my story, not just so you can get to know who I am, but so you can relate with the feelings and reactions I had while struggling to make a place in the world for my family. Our events and experiences will be different but we want the same things for our families though often we become lost and take the hardest road without realizing it. Keep reading to find yourself and find your way.

    Babies take a lot of time, energy, and patience. If you think you're busy and stressed out now, just wait—the addition of a screaming bundle of joy will give you more reasons to complain about how hectic life is and that you have no time for yourself, to wonder how you will pay for everything, how you will care for them, how you will react to braces and university, and to wonder whether they will look up to you.

STOP!

I want you to acknowledge the spinning in your head and that uncomfortable yet familiar feeling in your stomach. This is the exact perspective this book will help you shift. Pregnancy and parenthood are going to change every aspect of your life, and whether those changes will be positive or negative will be up to you. Working on the foundations of your health will help you find your truth and the assurance, strength, and clarity that comes with it.

Your child will enhance your life and open your eyes and heart in ways you never could have imagined. These gifts are automatically yours as a parent. But unless you allow yourself to be available to receive the gifts of fatherhood, intellectually, emotionally, spiritually, and physically, you will miss them and the window of opportunity is all too brief.

A strained relationship between you and your partner hurts both of you and is a negative model for your little one. Your child will look to you to learn about life, relationships, how to treat other people, and how to allow themself to be treated. Being an absent father—putting work first, turning to distractions such as television or drinks after work a little too often—is a loss of life for you and your family. You will rob them and yourself of the most important and wonderful gifts life has to offer, like the ache of joy in your chest watching your daughter skip away after giving you a hug. I'm not talking about the occasional event; I'm talking about being absent more often than not, even when you are physically present.

We have all seen the movies where the father is working hard trying to provide for his family, perhaps dealing with a dark past or childhood himself. He is focused on the promotion he needs to get, the deadline he needs to meet, or the payments he needs to make. The child is struggling, just trying to be seen. The child tries to show the drawing that he did of the family or to ask the father to come and watch his soccer game. We all want to shout at the screen, "LOOK AT WHAT'S RIGHT IN FRONT OF YOU." We want the father to be aware enough just to even notice.

Chapter 1

Well … this is your chance! This is your movie. For you to be in shape enough to give a horsey ride or a piggy back; to have the energy to engage with your family in a supportive rather than a reactive way. This is your chance to change your perspective to enhance your self-awareness so you are not the distracted father.

You may be noticing you have put on weight (fat). When you see an overweight father with an overweight child you may wonder, "How do I prevent that from happening to my child, when I can't stop it from happening to me?" I guarantee you if you follow what is laid out in these pages, you will come to know not only how to care for yourself, but how you will pass on the newly gained knowledge to your family.

Give yourself the strength and serenity that comes with knowing your priorities and allowing yourself to enjoy them. Be able to maintain your boundaries, not allowing yourself to be "pulled away." The important things are not the labels you are wearing, the car you are driving, or even the home you are living in. You know your truth; it is a knowledge that is inherent within all of us; it's just that we have been conditioned to think differently.

I did that—I thought differently. I went down the wrong path as a new father. I worked long hours trying to look good at work and provide a home with plenty of material things. But I went overboard, working too many hours, getting caught up in having "more."

The Roots of This Book

By the time my youngest son had arrived, I was so rarely at home that I was convinced when I was that he did not even like me (a great excuse to justify my lack of involvement). He would start to cry and look like he was panicking when I tried to play with him.

The fact was my son did not know me.

I could also see the uncertainty on the faces of my wife and daughter who did not know when I was going to leave and how to connect with me for the brief time I was at home.

Seeing the confusion and hurt my actions were creating led to even more pain and guilt, which in turn led to more justification for my actions leading to even more reactive behaviour on my part. I was in a vicious self-perpetuating cycle that gained momentum quickly.

Even when I was home, it was about what "I need to get done around the house." These were more avoidance strategies for what was really going on, not just with my family but with myself and my life.

I was so immersed and practised in my behaviours that I could not see they were what I was using to justify my dysfunctional coping mechanisms.

I came to a place where what I was doing was not working at all. In fact, I was destroying myself and hurting my family. What I was lacking could not be filled by nice stuff; I could not be helped by "more."

I came to that place not with my family but on the street; actually not even on the street—but in the alleys. The thing about damaging, coping mechanisms is they lead to the introduction of even more damaging (usually way more harmful), coping mechanisms. How that happens is by engaging in negative/reactive coping mechanisms, for example, anger. Anger sets a precedent, a new baseline, one that perpetuates the negative space, making self-harm easy to justify. The negativity continues with the guilt and shame that follow these reactive experiences.

The negative voice that was inside me allowed me to be more susceptible to ways of disconnecting and distracting: "Who cares if it's not good for me." I became more susceptible to things that I knew were not good for me. Creating a negative space makes executing negative behaviour much easier to do and to rationalize. I became more apt to listen when someone talked about what they "used" for stress or sleep or depression.

You can quickly—and without seeing or noticing it happen—end up in a place you could never have imagined. I know how that feels, like the world was pulled out from beneath my feet and all the air stolen from my lungs. A moment I will never forget and one I hope you never come to know. The thing is it works both ways: positive perception will lead to empowerment and happiness; negative perception will lead to misery. Either way has the potential to take you to places you would never have imagined. Perception is one of the most important things we have the ability to adjust.

I chased society's "carrot" and continued to mask the true emotions inside myself with reactive emotions like blame and anger. I used work and substances to create distraction and detachment from the truth of what was happening and what I was feeling.

I began to be surrounded by and drawn to those with the same negativity who were practising the same avoidance. This was definitely not a case of "strength in numbers"; it was more like "weakness more easily justified in numbers." It was a time when I would not have been able to understand that the opposite of courage is conformity. Conforming to what was around me seemed to be the choice I had to make, even though I could feel it was not a good choice. I understood my own conflict and my uneasy, uncertain feelings and to know that they were my truth trying to tell me to trust in what I knew was right. But I wasn't ready to live that truth yet.

Change occurred as it will in life but I was in a perpetual state of denial, constantly using negative perception. So the more I changed, the worse things got—everyone and everything else were the problems, according to my perspective.

I needed that perspective. Without it, I would have had to look at the truth and realize that my actions and reactions were the cause of my situation. I did not have the strength to even consider that at the time. The potential for (and even the notion of) hopeful change was so foreign I would not have known what to do or what the next step would even look like.

Guilt, hopelessness, confusion, fear, and overwhelming sadness were always with me. These feelings are important to discuss for they are shared by many people who lead "normal" lives and are not just the domain of the horrendously lost. Watch out for minimization. What I mean by "minimization" is the subtle depreciations we apply to ourselves. Contrived justification and rationalization collaborate with fear in not allowing us to be truthful with ourself about what we are feeling. A little sadness goes a long way. We don't need to get to the point where we are on our knees with no home, no money, no job, no food, no hope, our teeth clenched, with a tear-soaked face, yearning skyward, and growling for death.

I was and I can tell you with the utmost assuredness that I never want to be there again.

Oddly, that was not enough to elicit change, nor was the threat of losing my home, family, job, and life, all of which I did lose at one point or another on my journey. The threat or potential consequence of something negative is rarely a catalyst for positive change, but will instead always serve to perpetuate a fear-based life and continue negativity towards oneself and one's prospects.

After years of struggle, knowing I was lost and becoming more and more proficient at hating and harming myself, knowing I needed to get back to my family, the cycle of incarceration tipped the scale.

I had been in and out of being locked up, but the last time I was released, it happened that I had lost some of the connections to my familiar negative environment. I had lost touch with the circumstances and people who made it easier to ply my particular form of self-harm. I walked out of the detention centre with nowhere to go, wearing my prison release grey sweats and white Velcro sneakers. I had one bus ticket. I thought about selling it, but instead somehow I got on the bus. My mind was still telling me what it wanted, screaming chaos and negativity at me, constantly planning, blaming, justifying. Not having numbers to call or a place to find a familiar face (albeit of a negative acquaintance) were pivotal factors on my getting on that bus. I chose to not give myself the means to carry through on any of the negative thoughts or ideas that ran through my head. Instead, my heart-wrenching desire to be with my family was the push I needed. Being in a safe environment was the next critical step where expectations were limited, things were kept simple, and the burden of choice was removed from me. My penchant for the elaborate scenario was cut off; no more drama. There was no more leaving because "so and so was trying to kill me" or "I need to take care of such and such a scenario or I will go to prison." These could have been very real situations though; unless I allowed myself to let go, there would always be a "situation" to take care of. I was unable to access negative coping behaviours; nor was I able to be around other people living in a reactive and negative way. I stayed away from people who invested in and supported the burden and the spectacle.

It was not about making the "right choice." I did not at that time have the capacity to even know what that looked like, never mind actually to do it. I had developed my defense mechanisms and behaviours over a lifetime. I would feel and then react without thought; it was automatic.

So I gave myself permission not to know and to be open to new ways of seeing and being. In essence, I let go, a little at first, just sitting and trying not to "do" anything, just trusting the fact that my current internal processes and motivations were not helping me. I had trust in the framework I was being provided with, and I trusted that those supporting me had my and my family's best interests as their guidelines.

This situation left me more able to see my guiding light, my wife Shereesse. The noise and distraction I created for myself was so loud and encompassing I was hardly able to see her, never mind hear the common sense she was trying to give me. She had never given up on me and, setting up some strict boundaries, Shereesse gradually allowed me back into her inner circle.

Letting go in this way was both the hardest and the easiest thing I had ever done, though undoubtedly the best. It is from this letting go that new paths became available. I continue to grow and become happier to this day.

It is from this perspective that I created this book. Not from the "I know what I am doing" standpoint, but from the "I know what NOT to do" stance. Trust me. On this, I am an expert. This book is not merely about getting "ripped" abs or running a marathon, though this program absolutely lays the foundation and puts you on the path if those goals are on your horizon. This book is about finding out where you are, and then who you are.

This is what I am asking you to do: to let go, not in a grand gesture sort of way, but by keeping it simple, with the understanding that your current system may not be working in your best interest.

Remain mindful of the all-or-nothing mentality, which can be an effective way of setting yourself up for disappointment. So practise acceptance with no expectations, beginning with your physical connection and what you are putting in your body.

This is why I developed this book: to help other new dads find themselves and find their way, so we can become the change.

Becoming the change means leading by example, taking ownership of our lives and our perspectives, not living in fear and expectation, but with awareness and acceptance. This is important. As a father, we are responsible for the imprinting and development of our child in a very big way, through our actions, behaviours, and perceptions. If you can begin to identify the barriers and misconceptions you carry personally while staying involved and supportive of your partner during the pregnancy, it will be like having a running start for when the baby arrives.

This book is structured around the three trimesters of pregnancy and what you can expect to experience and what you can do to support your partner while finding yourself and applying the knowledge in this book. It is based on building a simple foundation of understanding and caring for yourself. It starts with what you put into your body and moves to identifying the negative little voice in your head that interferes in everything you do. This identification is critical so that when it comes to understanding and caring for your family, you will be ready and secure in the knowledge of your truth.

I can honestly say that the structure and practices laid out in this book are how I live on a daily basis. I am grateful to have them in my life and not just the belief in, but the knowledge of, their efficacy. I can easily say that if I had been following this program twenty-five years ago, things would have been way different for me, though I would not have had the challenges that have allowed me to gain this knowledge, the opportunity to pass it on, and the change to become the man and father I am today for which I am grateful. You could say it is a bit of a chicken-and-egg scenario. Well, I am providing you with the egg and you do not need to be chicken.

You may be wondering, "Why should I listen to this guy?" Well, I have been in the fitness community for thirty-five years. For twenty of those years, I was a trainer for many, including elite athletes, special need individuals, members of vulnerable populations, children, and seniors. I have a Human Kinetics Degree (B.H.K.) from the University of British Columbia. I am a professional natural bodybuilder and a Black Belt in Taekwondo. I am a Registered Canadian Art Therapist (RCAT) and I have practised my own personal growth, transformation, and recovery program for the last nine years; I continue to do so. I have been gifted with four beautiful children and two beautiful grandchildren. To top it all off, I am gloriously, happily married to the light of my life. I have and continue to apply everything you will read in this book. It is what I base my life on. I invite you to do the same.

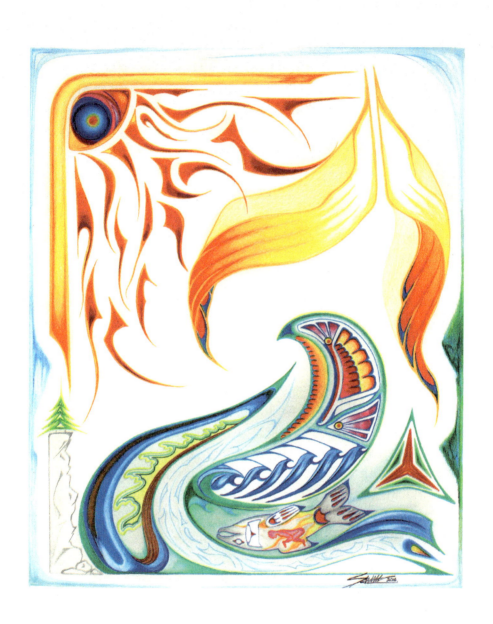

FIRST TRIMESTER

Chapter 2 Adrenalize Your Eating

Food is good; food keeps us alive. It nourishes our bodies and minds. It can bring us together and it can be creative and enjoyable. Food is not meant to be a way of avoiding or dealing with an emotional state and it absolutely should not make you feel bad or remorseful after you eat it.

Most of us developed a link between comfort and convenience food early in life. Did you go to McDonald's for family outings or to celebrate after the big game? Was getting pizza a special event? If you had a bad day, did your dad take you to Dairy Queen? Whatever the story, our brains form a link between these types of foods and emotional coping.

Unfortunately, most fast foods, convenience foods, and snack foods are not real food. They are food products that do not properly fuel our bodies and actually work against us. Eating junk food adds a rush of carbohydrates into our system. This rush of carbohydrates spikes our sugar levels and is quickly followed by a sugar low, wreaking havoc on our metabolism, our hormones, our thought processes, and our emotions. This actually causes us to become physically addicted.

Eating junk and fast food also creates a chemical imbalance in the brain. These foods are specifically designed to create a pleasure response: the refined sugar, salt, and fat—or various combinations of these—activate your brain to release endorphins, the same hormones linked to basic survival patterns like sex, love, attachment, and pain relief. These are the same patterns involved in drug addiction. Your processed food addiction is real with its connections running very deep.

According to a 2011 Bloomberg News story, Dr. Nora Volkow of the National Institute on Drug Abuse in the US says, "The data is so overwhelming the field has to accept it.... We are finding tremendous overlap between drugs in the brain and food in the brain."

Cocaine is something processed from the coca plant; heroin is something processed from poppies; sugar is something processed from sugar cane; high fructose corn syrup is something processed from corn. We have taken these naturally occurring substances and intensified their concentrations to grossly unnatural levels, which causes our bodies to have grossly unnatural responses. This leads to us seeking out this quick fix through external coping mechanisms. And we wonder why we are all losing touch with our inherent coping mechanisms, our strength, and our sense of what food is and what it is meant to do!

In 2007, a French experiment showed that cocaine-addicted rats preferred water sweetened with saccharine or sugar to cocaine.

The depths and effect of our food sources upon us combined with the titanic amount of deliberate manipulation and alteration performed by the food industry is just starting to be brought out in the open.

If you find yourself saying, "C'mon, I'm not addicted to junk or processed food," then I challenge you to eat the way I suggest here. If you cannot do that for three months (heck, try it for a week), you need to seriously look at the "reasons" (your excuses) why you can't eat the way we are designed to. You will never find your truth unless you are first honest with yourself.

Junk food products hurt your body. Because junk food and snacks are usually high in empty calories and low in nutrients, your body doesn't feel satisfied, and doesn't send your brain the "Full, stop eating" signal. As mentioned earlier the processing of our foods causes extreme concentrations of "flavour" that stimulate abnormal hormone response not only in the body but in the brain as well.

In a 2010 study carried out by the University of Texas and the

Oregon Research Institute, twenty-six overweight young women were given magnetic resonance imaging (MRI) scans as they sipped a milkshake made with Haagen-Dazs ice cream and Hershey Co.'s chocolate syrup. Six months later, the same women had repeat MRI scans. Those who had gained weight showed reduced activity in the striatum (a region of the brain that registers reward), when they sipped milkshakes the second time. These results were published in the *Journal of Neuroscience*.

"A career of overeating causes blunted reward receipt, and this is exactly what you see with chronic drug abuse," said Eric Stice, researcher at the Oregon Research Institute.

People addicted to processed foods end up eating more than if they were to eat real food. And, those empty sugars, fats, and artificial calories go right into fat storage.

Think about it this way: you have a choice of two kinds of gas for your car. Gas A will make your car run like crap—blowing gaskets, clogging up fuel lines, backfiring—and you'll have to take your car for repairs all the time, until your mechanic (whose new boat you paid for) tells you it's no longer worth fixing.

Gas B, on the other hand, will make your car perform like a Formula One machine, greatly increase its lifespan with no trips to the shop, and make it look like a Ferrari.

Which gas would you choose? It's a no-brainer, right? You know what to put in a car. But what kind of fuel are you putting in your body?

An article in the *American Journal of Medicine* reports on a study that adopted a holistic approach to determine the association of diet with overall health at older ages. The researchers examined whether diet (assessed in midlife using what and when the participants ate and how closely they followed the Alternative Healthy Eating Index (AHEI)) changes our body size and shape as we get older. Individuals participated sixteen years on average. Five thousand, three hundred and fifty adults aged between forty-five and fifty-six were assessed every five years. The less individuals stuck to the AHEI, the higher were the risks of death from all kinds of illnesses. People in the study who ate a North American diet of processed foods, sweets, white flour, red meat, and high-fat dairy had lower odds of ideal aging, no matter what else they were doing like playing sports, working out, yoga, etc.

Basically, living on the "Western diet" is a horrible way to grow old and die. To combat this, you need to start to move more. If you begin to exercise regularly—and even if you do nothing else—you will turn on and speed up your body's metabolism, giving it a reason to come alive and creating somewhere for all that food to go. Of course, as you do this one thing, you will create an environment of increased wellness. This is a great momentum to perpetuate and it will lead to awareness in other areas.

There is no reason for us to be eating processed foods; these food products are food substitutes. They are created to create a market, not to feed the body. The problem is that they've become so accepted and integrated into our lives that no one even questions them. Well now, it's time to stop and ask some questions.

Every time you eat, ask yourself, "Is this feeding my body?" If the answer is no, then what is it feeding and why are you putting it in your mouth? Remember this is not about denying yourself or beating yourself up. This is only about raising awareness around why you eat what you eat; finding out what's really going on inside

Do not, I repeat, DO NOT be negative on yourself—that negativity will not serve you. In fact, it will only reinforce poor eating habits. A negative self-perception is an easy "go to" and a familiar place for some as it is used on a daily basis by most people in modern society to justify inappropriate behaviours, reactions, self-serving perceptions, detrimental consumption, and let's not forget lethargy. A negative self-perception creates the environment in which doing something to yourself that you know is not good for you is easy, possibly even seen as deserved.

As you go through the trials and challenges of change, try instead to increase your self-awareness, remaining open nonjudgmentally to learning what the circumstances were that activated the true underlying emotions, which in turn activated the reactionary response.

By asking yourself questions, you acknowledge yourself, and you help to identify your behaviours. This makes you vastly increase your self-awareness. This new perspective will give you the opportunity to say, "Hey, why the heck am I doing this to myself?" You may already have an idea as to why. The big difference between continuing in ignorance and becoming self-aware is you are no longer immersed in the behaviour and the emotion. This new stance allows you to catch your breath and be in the present. Now, through increased awareness, you are in a position to do something about the negative behaviour, if you decide it is something you would like to do, also allowing you to step out of the emotion and become more firmly in the present.

This is how you empower yourself and begin to identify the areas you would like to alter. You have the ability to break the cycle of bad eating that has been handed down through as many as even four generations. In doing so, you will become the change for your little one who is on the way.

The Adrenaline Factor

You need to get ready for the physical, mental, and emotional demands of fatherhood. This is where the Adrenaline Factor comes in. It's a workout and a nutrition philosophy that's perfect for a new dad, and a great start to a strong family.

The Adrenaline Factor workout is the result of what I've learned from thirty-plus years in the fitness industry. I've worked and studied with old-school power lifters, modern body sculptors, martial arts experts, and academic scholars. I've seen what worked, and more importantly, learned from what wasn't as effective. I developed this workout so you can gain maximum fitness in minimum time without harming your body. It's a new way of thinking that focuses on identification, acceptance, and progressive change, which means meeting your needs and your schedule.

The Adrenaline Factor is not just another routine—it's a formula for life and the difference between suffering through it or living it.

- Your body will become leaner, with less body fat.
- You'll be stronger and more muscular.
- You'll have more energy—a real bonus for new dads!
- You'll feel calmer and have better coping mechanisms.
- You'll sleep better and wake up feeling refreshed.
- Your libido will increase, and your body's physical response to intimate stimulus will also improve (think Viagra without the Viagra).
- Tightening things up will help you feel more desirable and confident.
- Overall, you will be happier.

The Adrenaline Factor philosophy gives you an easy-to-follow start and keeps the improvements coming. By using the Adrenaline Factor for three months, you will lose fat, gain muscle, and have more energy. The quick simple workouts will leave you feeling energized, relaxed, and you will be better able to focus on enjoying your new family.

Knowledge is power only if you apply it and I'm here to show you the way. Anyone can toss you a few trout, but I am here to teach you how to fish. By explaining the Adrenaline Factor philosophy and workout and by explaining the best ways to support your pregnant partner, *Fit for Fatherhood* will

- Enhance your food knowledge and how to eat to get the results you want.

- Show you an easy-to-start progressive workout that gives maximum results in minimum time.
- Give you tips on building a stronger relationship. I'll tell you what's going on with your partner during each trimester of her pregnancy and I'll explain how to support her as you prepare for the adventure ahead.
- Explain what you can expect to be feeling yourself, supplying you with some tools to use to keep you involved and feel grounded.
- Promote balance, structure, and awareness in all other aspects of your life.

Following the program will give you the energy and vitality to pursue an active and involved life with your partner and children. It will also give you knowledge to pass on to your children. The most important type of knowledge there is is the knowledge of your own truth. Developing this knowledge will allow you and your family to more easily recognize what your priorities are. It will also provide protection against the onslaught of external stressors socially, spiritually, mentally, and economically. Your family will have a strong foundation to stand upon, so you can make decisions clearly and simply, ensuring a bright and healthy future for them and their future loved ones.

Why Counting Calories Is Not Ideal for Improving Fitness

The traditional method for losing weight was taking in fewer calories—the old calorie count. Unfortunately, that method tends to be very stressful and does not address the reality of what is going on for you. There are many reasons why I say this, and I will mention a couple.

I can think of few things more laborious or off-putting than figuring out the calorie content of every item on your plate at every meal.

Restriction and the feeling of denial is probably, for most, one of the main reasons for inappropriate consumption. I know if I tell myself I can't have something it's usually the first thing I want!

Common misperceptions are "I feel depressed; maybe I need anti-depressants; if I only won the lottery, everything would be better; I'm too fat; I need to be on a diet." This type of thinking is symptom-based reactive analysis or quick-fix problem-solution mentality. By adrenalizing your eating, we are going further to the foundation, asking what type of food is going into our bodies and wondering whether it is food at all. This questioning will affect all aspects of our wellness. Understanding the type of calories you are ingesting will help with your food choices. The *type* of calories you get are immensely more important than their quantity. This can also become very complex and confusing.

It's important to understand the quality of the calories you consume rather than consider counting how many are going in. For example, are you eating processed or whole foods? What's their fat and protein content, fibre, artificial ingredients, etc.?

What Do I Mean by Adrenalizing Your Eating?

The Adrenaline Factor looks beyond calories or rather, before calories, simplifying not complicating things. It brings us back to a foundational perspective that is simple and powerful; I call it "adrenalizing." By adrenalizing your eating, you build and tone your muscle mass to fire up your metabolism. Your metabolism is the speed at which you convert your food to the building blocks your body requires; it's how your body utilizes the food you eat and breaks it down to use its constituents at the cellular level for building and repairing tissue and organs. It is also responsible for energy creation and storage. By adrenalizing your eating, you change the way you burn fat and store glycogen. Glycogen is the fuel stored in your muscles, which we not only use in the gym but when we get up from our chair or run up a flight of stairs. It is stored in the muscles in only limited amounts.

Adrenalizing your eating is about eating real food that fuels your body, and that your body knows what to do with. It's about simplifying your eating and allowing your body to find its balance.

Adrenalizing your eating is taking responsibility and empowering yourself. It's not about being told what to do—it's knowing what to do and doing it. It's about accepting and taking care of yourself, which in turn allows you to accept and support the ones you love.

Don't spend your day thinking about things you can't do or things you should have done. Spend your days doing. Chapter 4 will provide the details and some more very relevant information for you to feel good about adrenalizing.

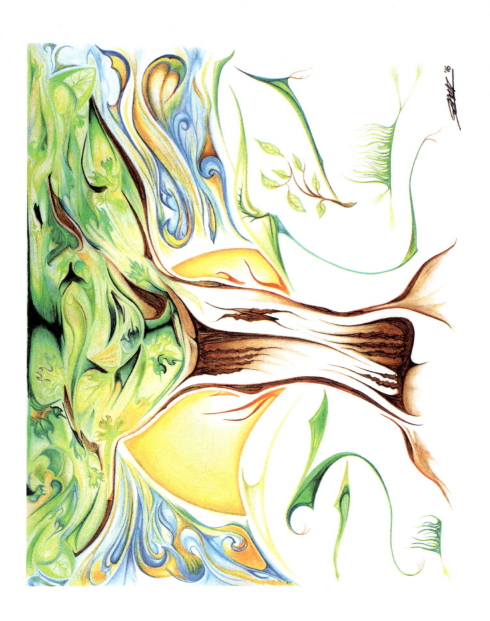

Chapter 3 The Phase 1 Workout

Your partner has already embarked on her journey and has been working away physically, emotionally, and mentally creating life. That's right; it's time for you to do something awesome too. The good news is we are going to start off well within your ability and with awareness rather than expectation. Phase 1 is a reintroduction to your body. We're going to reactivate your muscles, clear out the neuromuscular connections, and reteach your body how to position itself. In this phase I want you to pay close attention to maintaining correct body posture to maximize your workout's efficiency, effectiveness, and safety. You will be developing body awareness; creating a foundation for continuing to learn how to move properly, and learning how your body and muscles feel when you do.

The psychological part of Phase 1 is accepting that you're just starting. Don't try to rush the process. Heighten your awareness around self-judgment when you compare yourself to others or to where you used to be. Recognize self-judgment as your critic, the ugly voice that gets in our way; we hear it but do not listen. This is a voice we want to get to know. Every time it speaks, put it where you can see it and then let it go and move forward. This is your journey and the fact that you are even thinking about getting *Fit for Fatherhood* puts you at a new level of opportunity.

Before getting started, relax somewhere, and consider the reasons you are beginning this journey. Take a picture of yourself, shirt off, acknowledging yourself and listening for the negative voice. Print out the photo and, on the back, write your goals. Write down anything else you are feeling or thinking; this will be relevant later in your journey. On a separate piece of paper, put down your reasons for creating these goals and put them where you will see them, allowing them to speak to you every day. This process will help create your launching pad, providing you with a solid foundation from which you can take your first step with acknowledgement and understanding of your reasons, a fence around the vulnerability of your truth to help combat the critic.

Accepting your starting level will help you when it comes to the exercises. It will allow you to create an authentic starting point, setting you up for solid progressive growth. We live in a society in which we are busy trying to get, be, or go somewhere—so busy trying to get "there," that we're not "here." Allow yourself to be in the moment, being present in whatever you are doing, be it a squat press, writing a report, or listening to your partner. The Adrenaline Factor is built on easy, progressive change, and may feel too easy at first, but if you allow the exercises to be new and pay attention to following correct Foundational Form, you will quickly develop good movement routines.

By allowing yourself not to be proficient, you will soon become proficient. Finding your authentic origin and consistently applying sound principles will provide progressive transformation.

You don't need to bust your butt every time—or any of the time for that matter. You are meant to do the routines at your own level of comfort, which means it's okay to vary them from day to day. Just doing the routine will create positive and progressive change, developing a shift in perspective around prioritizing self-care. Keep things at your own pace and intensity level, while being mindful of what you're doing and how you feel.

I don't want you to turn your workouts into a form of self-harm. You may already be heaping expectation on yourself. Self-harm takes many shapes, from behavioural addictions like substance abuse, workaholism, and food addiction, to self-denial, anger, and negative self-image. Our negative voice most often works in very indirect and complex ways, taking many forms, all of them toxic.

Stop trying to get more; allow yourself to become more.

The physical nature of working out can be a great way of acknowledging emotions and working through them. It is important to stay honest and present with yourself. This will allow your physiologically and psychologically inherent processes to work, letting the stresses of the mind and body dissipate. Getting angry as you work out—whether it's at yourself for the shape you're in, your day at work, the guys talking too loudly next to you—is a way of distracting and externalizing, making something positive into a torture session. Being able to stay present with yourself will empower you in your workout. Practise staying present and aware of yourself in your workouts so you can get to know how to do it effectively and apply it to other circumstances and areas of your life.

Before we get started, I want to take a moment to talk about some of the mental barriers to building a successful fitness routine. Don't let these common inaccuracies in thinking distract you from your commitment to lasting health:

This Is Too Easy!

When you first start a workout program, the burn or "pump" will not be as intense. The muscle burn or pump when you exercise is a feeling you will become familiar with if you are not already. Do not worry. This is normal and a good sign that you are working a particular muscle. It is what is called "lactic acid build up" in the muscle and it will clear out as soon as you stop exercising. This is normal. You may not have been exercising those muscles in a while, so the veins, vessels, and neural pathways to, in, and around those areas have been underutilized. Be careful not to misinterpret this and think, "Hey, I'm in better shape than I thought" or "I don't feel anything" and go harder. Going harder inevitably ends up in the next three days being very painful. This is not only a physical kick in the butt, it also creates a huge mental barrier. Instead of thinking, "Boy, I can't wait to do that again," you'll be muttering, "Not bloody likely." This leaves a negative connection to exercise and anything resembling it. This can diminish momentum and give the negative voice an opportunity to put its foot in the door.

For the first week, at least wait until the second day after the exercises to assess the intensity or weights used. The best case scenario at this point would be to use no weights. It will take time (more time than you might think) to even start to see how prevalent our critic (our ego) is once we start to add a value to anything (in this case, weights). The weights we will be using here are quite light; five pounds will probably be adequate in most cases. The resistance should be light enough so the emphasis is on strict technique and feeling the muscle move. I suggest at first to not use any weight and move your body only through the exercise. This is to gain familiarity with the movement for your mind and your body, thereby enhancing the neuromuscular and cardiovascular pathways for the movement.

If you work out on Monday, Wednesday will be the day you have the greatest muscle soreness. Remember, eating and sleeping effectively will reduce the length and severity of LOMS (latent onset muscle soreness).

This Is Too Easy! (Part 2)

Another misconception about exercise is that your routine should be exhausting—that you need to push your body to the limit every time. This is just not true. Your body is made to move, run, and play, and your workouts should be an enjoyable part of your daily maintenance. If you are moving at your own pace, you will enjoy your workout and find it easier to maintain your new lifestyle. Stimulate; don't annihilate.

It's Been a Week—Shouldn't I Be Fit by Now?

Most people do not get to enjoy progress with their fitness because their workouts are focused on unrealistic end goals and short time frames rather than on awareness and consistency. Frequently diets and workouts are designed for big gains in a short time. These are stressful physically and mentally, intense and restrictive, making them nearly impossible and unhealthy to maintain for any significant amount of time. This is a great way to keep confused and unbalanced—what the diet and weight-loss industry counts on! Having a goal is not a bad thing—goals motivate and guide us—but a pass or fail mentality causes you to miss the journey, which in this case, is your life.

The Ghost of Exercise Past

I would lay odds that you have worked out before—that you set fitness goals and invested in equipment or a gym membership. Maybe you were successful for a while, or maybe the equipment turned into a clothes rack. You probably achieved some fitness but not the level you'd like. For whatever reason, the workout stalled and your hope was replaced with other distractions.

What roadblocks have you experienced when you've tried to start a workout program? Do any of these sound familiar?

- I didn't make the time.
- I am too busy at work or school.
- I'll start next month or after the holidays.
- I only went when I felt like it and I never felt like it.
- I'm so out of shape, I don't know where to start.
- I didn't like the gym or the trainer.
- I felt out of place.
- It's too hard on my back/knees/body.
- I hated the activities I was doing.
- I'm not a fitness guy.
- I didn't get the results I was looking for.

- My schedule changed and I just never got back into it.
- I hated the way I looked in workout gear.
- I was getting too big or bulky looking.
- I had an injury or accident.
- I couldn't afford it.

Imagine which roadblocks you'll face this time. Lack of time is a common one for most people, never mind for new parents (what I designed this program around)! See if you can come up with a solution to each roadblock before it arises. For example, if you feel out of place in the gym, you could go at a different time or find another gym. Can't afford a gym? Use the big free one outside. You need to make yourself and your health a priority. This program is designed to be done anywhere from your office to your living room.

If your problem is getting up for a morning workout, make sure your alarm is loud or try standing ankle-deep in ice water for twenty seconds (just cold water will do). Either of these methods will shock your nervous system, giving it an immediate rush of energy. I go with an old standby—a cup of coffee before I start does the trick for me.

This program's time requirement is designed to fit any schedule, so if you are having trouble getting started you need to remove the option of not doing it. Commit to a workout partner or agree to start the program at the same time with someone. You can both be going to the same gym or across the country if you are in contact and supporting each other positively, watching each other's back. We are just talking about the workout; he does not need to be expecting also. So if you have a friend who has been struggling to make a change, now may be the time to do it together. Making yourself accountable to someone else helps you follow through, and builds support and motivation at the same time. Remember that you are having a child. When you have trouble staying positive for yourself, doing it for someone else is a great way to have it mirrored back to you.

Get a dog. Researchers have found that people who own dogs walk almost twice as much as those without. Can't have a dog? Lots of humane societies and SPCAs appreciate volunteer dog walkers. Or just take yourself for a walk!

Prepare. Use mental imaging to put yourself in the time and place when you will be working out. Professional athletes have used this technique for decades to prepare for big games and tough opponents. Imagine what you are going to do and how it will feel, right down to the last detail. Rehearse it in your mind before you start so when the moment comes you will be ready and committed. This technique can also be used to prepare for any of life's challenging events from public speaking to speaking with your partner.

Once you slay the excuse dragon, you're ready to meet motivational challenges head-on. This will make your life easier: instead of worrying about what excuse to use or feeling guilty for using it, you'll be into your workout before even thinking of it as optional.

The Foundational Form for All Exercises

Now we're going to get active. Remember that body posture and control are essential! The following is a list of instructions for the basic body position for all the exercises, not only in this program but for anything you are doing from walking down the street to sitting in a chair. I recommend you practise this position and maintain body awareness around it as much as you can.

- Head in a neutral position in line with your spine
- Shoulders back and down (palms of your hands should be at your sides)
- Chest up
- Knees slightly bent (not locked)
- Butt out and tight (maintaining the curve in your lower back)

- Abdominals engaged (sucked in)

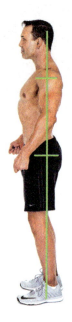 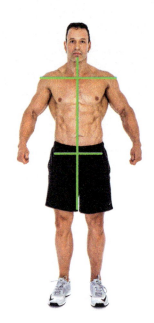

Do not twist or curl your body during the exercises. Twisting or rounding decreases the efficiency of the exercises. Keep your body square with the axis of rotation and do not bend but fold and rotate at the hips and shoulders trying not to curl your back or shoulders.

Maintaining this posture during exercise means that your muscles and tendons will develop and support your body naturally in its strongest position.

Never sacrifice proper form for speed or weight. Do what you can while maintaining proper form.

If you try to do too much or go too fast, the beneficial effects of your movements will decrease and your risk of injury will increase.

What we are doing now is creating a foundation regarding teaching and strengthening your body in its optimal anatomical position.

Reps and Sets

"Reps" is short for "repetitions" of exercises. It means the number of times to perform the movement from start to finish. For example, "Reps: 12 push-ups" means do 12 push-ups. Starting in the "up" position, lowering to the floor, and pushing back up to the starting "up" position is one rep.

When you have done the prescribed reps for an exercise, you've completed 1 Set. Three sets of twelve or 3x12 push-ups would be three groups of twelve reps.

JUST FOR TODAY

Monday

> **NEVER SACRIFICE PROPER FORM FOR SPEED OR WEIGHT! DO WHAT YOU CAN WHILE MAINTAINING PROPER FORM.**

10-Minute Morning Shot of Adrenaline

When: before breakfast

Reps

12 jumping jacks
12 step-ups with exaggerated arm movements
12 ball punch crunches
Perform 12 reps of each of the 3 exercises as many times as you can in 10 minutes, resting as little as possible. Push yourself and do them as fast as you can while still maintaining proper form.

20-Minute Body Sculpting

When: anytime during the day
Reps
20 squats with press
10 per side: wide leg plank with one arm pull
30 step-ups
20 push-ups (if you can't do regular push-ups, put your knees on the floor).

Perform 3 sets within the 20-minute period with minimal to no rest time between exercises. After completing the 4 exercises, that is one set. Rest no more than 2 minutes and have some water between sets. If you cannot finish 3 sets within the 20-minute period, cut the reps in half for each exercise. If you find it easy, do as many sets as you can within the 20-minute period.

Exercise Details

As I said above, the Adrenaline Factor focuses on your posture and body position as you move. This makes all the difference in the results you will see. When I do these workouts with a client, I lay out the exercises and the pictures on the floor for reference. Because I'm not with you, I've compiled them all alphabetically in Appendix A at the back. Please refer to that right now.

JUST FOR TODAY

Rest Day

A rest day can mean something different for everyone as you might imagine. In the Adrenaline Factor, it means a less intense day in addition to the balanced structure in the rest of the workout. It is a day to stretch, play a sport, do some yoga, or have a picnic at the park.

Tuesday

10-Minute Morning Shot of Adrenaline

When: before breakfast

Reps

15 each leg running on the spot with knees high
12 squat punches
12 push ups (on knees is okay; maintain form)

Perform 12 reps of each of the 3 exercises as many times as you can in 10 minutes, resting as little as possible. Push yourself and do them as fast as you can while still maintaining proper form. Refer to Appendix A for details of all the exercises.

For Today

You may feel a little tight today so walk to the store or around the block and as you are watching television tonight, sit on the floor for at least 15 minutes and do some light stretching.

Stretching is a fantastic way to get in tune with your body. Stretching increases your health and fitness, and decreases your soreness and risk of injury.

Some stretches for today: hamstring, quads, and triceps. Refer to Appendix B for details of all the stretches.

Wednesday

10-Minute Morning Shot of Adrenaline

When: before breakfast

Reps

12 forearm extensions on the ball on knees
12 hold side-to-side jumps on toes with arms out
12 guarding stance with leg switch

Do as many sets as you can in 10 minutes, resting as little as possible. Push yourself and go as fast as you can while maintaining proper form.

20-Minute Body Sculpting

When: anytime during the day

Reps

20 straight leg deadlift with press
10 each side: one-arm ball rows
20 each side: lunges
10 push-ups to plank

Perform 3 sets within 20 minutes. If you find this easy, do as many sets as you can in the 20 minutes. If you can't finish 3 sets in 20 minutes, do half the number of reps for each exercise. Rest up to 2 minutes and drink water between sets.

Thursday

Rest Day

10-Minute Morning Shot of Adrenaline

When: before breakfast

Reps

15 fast feet
15 lunges

Do as many sets as you can in 10 minutes, resting as little as possible. Push yourself and go as fast as you can while maintaining proper form. Keep yourself active on your rest days. Park a couple of blocks away from where you are going. You will feel refreshed and ready to go when you reach your destination.

Some stretches for today: back, glutes, triceps, glute and back.

Friday

10-Minute Morning Shot of Adrenaline

When: before breakfast

Reps

10 jumping jacks
10 push-ups
10 squat punches

Do as many sets as you can in 10 minutes, resting as little as possible. Push yourself and go as fast as you can while maintaining proper form.

20-Minute Body Sculpting

When: anytime during the day

Reps

15 squats with curl
5 chair dips
5 per side: push pull push-ups
10 bike abs

Perform 3 sets within 20 minutes. If you find this easy, do as many sets as you can in the 20 minutes. If you can't finish 3 sets in 20 minutes, do half the number of reps for each exercise. Rest up to 2 minutes and drink water between sets.

Chapter 3

Saturday

10-Minute Morning Shot of Adrenaline

When: before breakfast

Reps

20 sets of Body Wake-Up

Today's morning shot of adrenaline is slightly different. This is one set:

Stand with your hands on your hips. Squat until your thighs are parallel to the floor, then raise back up to standing position. If you are a little tight at the start, either go as far as you can maintaining form or widen your stance.

With your legs straight touch your quads, knees, shins, or toes, whichever your start point may be. (Do not curl your back).

Keeping your legs straight, come back up to standing position.

Keeping your arms straight lift them above your head and then back down to your hips.

Plan an activity outside the home even if it's just going to the grocery store or walking around the mall. Start getting used to planning an activity.

Sunday

10-Minute Morning Shot of Adrenaline

When: before breakfast

Reps

20 jumping jacks
15 guarding stance with leg switch

Do at least 3 sets, followed by some easy stretching. This is a lighter day, but this little bit of activity will keep your body limber and help you maintain the workout flow.

Spend an hour minimum doing something active indoors or outdoors with your partner. It can be as simple as putting out the blanket and rolling a ball back and forth.

Fear and distrust produce reaction.
Purpose and truth produce action.

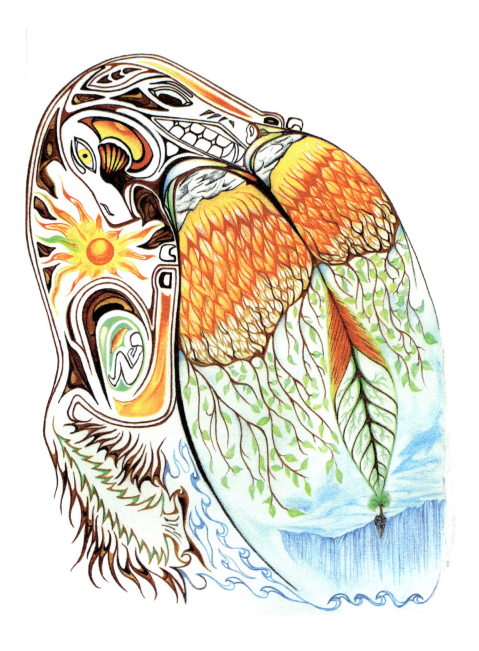

Chapter 4 Supporting Your Partner in the First Trimester

You're going to be a father, wow! I bet it seemed surreal when you first got the news. Don't worry—that surreal feeling will soon be replaced by fear and panic. These feelings are normal and good signs that you are going to be a great father. This is where the awareness we have been working on will help stop our minds from taking off to "what if" land, where things can quickly become very stressful. Absolutely the best things you can do here are to let go, live in the moment, and allow yourself to enjoy this precious time.

Hold your partner and see the happiness in her eyes and allow her to see your happiness. What she needs right now is to know that you will be there for her and that she has and always will have your support. She may look happy and in control, but she has her own worries, like losing her shape, having a unhealthy baby, the pain of childbirth … the list goes on. Now is the time to be by her side as you begin your journey to parenthood together.

4 Things You Can Do to Strengthen Your Role in the Pregnancy

Get a Notebook/ A Shelf/ A Drawer/ A Box

This will be your pregnancy journal. In it, you will keep pregnancy-related names, phone numbers, book titles, and other information.

Add your doctors' contact information, important dates, and emerging plans. Some people prefer to do this digitally using project management software or social media. Use whatever works for you; just make sure you have a central place for all the information that's coming your way.

Go to the Doctor

Unless your regular doctor delivers babies, one of the first things you need to do is find an obstetrician, a midwife, or other licensed childbirth professional.

How do you find a doctor who is right for you? Just like you'd get three quotes on a renovation job or before buying a fridge, shop around for a medical caregiver. There are lots of options here, so take time to research each style before choosing the one who best suits you and your partner. Ask friends, family, and co-workers who are parents, "Do you have some recommendations or tips?"

Set up interview meetings with potential caregivers and pick the one you and your partner are most comfortable with. These questions might help you decide.

- How easy was it to contact the office?
- How long did you have to wait for the appointment? What are their normal wait times?
- Is the receptionist friendly, patient, and understanding? (You will be dealing with him/her a lot, so this will become important.)
- Is the doctor friendly or distracted?
- Do they treat you and your partner with respect?
- Do they fully answer your questions using words that you understand?
- Do they downplay your concerns or make you feel less-than?
- Do they support the kind of birth you want—at home, in a hospital, etc.?

- What are their backup plans if they're not available for appointments or for the birth?
- Will they be able to continue being your child's doctor after your child is born? Do they provide care for babies and children?

Go to the Doctor Again

Your partner will probably see her caregiver regularly throughout the pregnancy. Usually it's monthly at first, then more frequently near the end. Always make the time to go with her, even if she says you don't have to. Be there for support—you are her champion and the person who is always on her side making sure she is safe, comfortable, and understands what's going on. Imagine her sitting by herself in the waiting room and the other mothers-to-be are there with their partners … you get the idea. And be there for yourself—hearing your baby's heartbeat for the first time is an experience you don't want to miss.

Be Involved at the Appointment

Just because your partner is the one getting checked over doesn't mean you can't or shouldn't be involved. It's up to you to look out for your partner and see what she may not see. She may feel apprehensive or may not want to rock the boat. Her body is releasing huge amounts of hormones and these do affect the way the brain works so she may not be thinking or remembering as she usually does. Discuss this with your partner before you go into the appointment so you can be on the same page as much as possible. Check that she is comfortable with your asking questions and share what you may be thinking of asking. Have a look or a signal for "be quiet" or "not now." In my case, my wife had a "what the #*&% is wrong with you?" look; she still uses it to this day; admittedly, I give her ample reason to use it.

You both will have lots of questions, and answering your questions is part of your doctor's job. Take time to make sure you understand and are satisfied with the answers. If you don't, ask for a translation: "explain it to me slowly"; or ask for it to be simplified: "explain it like I was five." Write everything down: questions, answers, new words, what has happened, what might happen—everything. Don't be worried about looking uncertain or like you don't know what's going on. Watch out for that false ego and the unrealistic expectation your inner critic puts on you. You are responsible for a little life now; the more involved you make yourself, the more you will feel a part of the process.

Before the appointment: Make a list of all the questions you want to ask, especially the ones your partner may feel uncomfortable asking. Don't be shy—your doctor has heard it all before. You can also ask for extra resources like books, websites, or apps. Go over your list before the appointment to make sure you've included all of your concerns and questions.

At the appointment: Bring your notebook and write down any answers or instructions. Writing down the answers helps you understand them and creates a personalized pregnancy resource and journal. If you are on the ball and recording things like answers, times, and dates, the doctor will notice. By doing your due diligence, you will automatically hold the doctor to a higher degree of accountability. By raising the level of your game, you will inspire those around you to do the same.

What She's Going Through: 10 Common First Trimester Experiences

1. **Tender breasts**: Be careful not to bump into them and handle them with care.
2. **Nausea**: Pregnancy can cause nausea and vomiting anytime

of the day or night; it's often referred to as Morning Sickness. There are ways to help her by keeping dry crackers—or other foods that appeal to her—nearby. Make sure you check what she wants because pregnancy hormones can change her tastes almost overnight; even if something was a favourite last week, this week it may literally make her sick. This is a common experience in pregnancy—she's not just being fussy.

3. **Sensitivity to smell, taste, touch**: All her senses will be heightened, like the alien in *Species*. (And she may be just as dangerous!) This heightened sensitivity will have a direct and rapid effect on her nausea.
4. **Intense food cravings**: Sometimes this translates into crazy combinations like pickles and ice cream or extreme levels of protein such as burgers, ham, steak, or cheese. Reminding her about possible weight gain is not helpful and potentially catastrophic!
5. **Insatiable hunger**: Try and remember how you were as a teenager, then get out of her way.
6. **Fatigue**: Energy levels may vary but tend to be low. She may feel sleepy and sluggish.
7. **Low sex drive**: Not much interest now, but that will change!
8. **Moodiness**: Hormones create different moods. Her moods may be affected by fears and worries. Sometimes they may not seem rational, but don't try to fix them; be supportive in the moment.
9. **Irritability**: Her patience may not be as per normal. She may be finding it difficult to be as patient as she would normally like to be.
10. **Excited/shocked/fearful**: Even if all goes well, she may be distracted with worries about the future and her abilities as a mother.

Improve Your Communication

Pregnancy is a time of increased and enhanced emotions—hope, excitement, fear, and worry—and your partner's changing hormones will affect her moods in ways that may seem strange. This is a time when good communication can really strengthen your relationship.

Good communication is not just how you listen but how you look when you listen.

You need to identify what you are feeling, not only for yourself but for her too. You also need to discuss what you are feeling with your partner. If you go around as if you are unaffected, it may seem as though you don't care. Lose the stiff-upper-lip mentality; if you keep your feelings inside, they will fester and show up later as inappropriate reactions. She needs to know what is affecting you positively or negatively. Share your feelings, leading the way for her to do the same.

Be her sounding board. Listen to her. Let her talk. I know you want to fix her problems and protect her, but what she really needs is to be heard and supported. Recognizing our emotions is the most important step in coping. We must allow them to do what they were meant to do: to allow life events and challenges to become part of our story and part of our strength.

Our emotions are our guides; when we do not acknowledge them we become lost.

Let her know you value her feelings, opinions, knowledge, and experience. The more you know about what is going on in her life, the more you can do to help, even if it's just by being there. Good communication will help you have a better understanding for when to stick around and when she needs space.

This is a time when friends and relatives can overdo it in the attention and advice department, so be there for her support. Be prepared to step in and change the conversation if she is becoming overwhelmed or suggest a time to catch up at a later date. Offer a back rub or a foot massage after the visit to allow her to decompress and voice any concerns.

Be a Gentleman

If you have been together for some time, the niceties may have diminished somewhat since your first date. You have become comfortable and familiar with each other. Now is the perfect time to brush up on those small acts that show you care and are paying attention.

This is your chance to step in and truly be a helping hand while at the same time making her feel like the special person she is. All the polite manners you learned over the years have very practical applications for protecting your partner's physical and emotional wellbeing now. Injuries can happen anytime, but during pregnancy she must be especially careful. Opening doors, carrying the groceries, and taking her arm across a slippery floor or upstairs are practical ways to safeguard your family.

When walking through a crowded mall, take her by the hand and lead the way to protect her from bumping or tripping. Remember to walk at a pace that's comfortable for her.

If you have to wait in line, find a seat for her while you stay in line.

Answer the phone for her and take messages when she's too tired to talk.

Make sure there isn't a constant stream of visitors invading your space. (That stream will become a river once the baby arrives, so now is your chance to practise being the bouncer.)

Lead by Example

We as men, fathers, and fathers-to-be must be responsible for the example we set and influence we create. You have always been responsible for the results of your own actions, but now the consequences also affect your family. Your actions will play a major role in the development and shaping of behaviours and perspectives for your new family. As you take this opportunity to reset and adjust your life for the better, there are certain behaviours which you must identify, acknowledge and reassess.

- **Alcohol**: if you can't stop drinking for nine months, you have identified a behaviour that is in the way of your happiness.
- **Smoking**: of any kind. Bringing anything to your mouth that is deleterious to your wellness is a good reason to raise your awareness around it. This type of activity also leaves toxic residue on your clothes, skin, and environment, which can be transferred to others who come in contact with it.
- **Eating high-fat and fried foods**: They're not good for either of you.
- **Caffeine**: Don't drink it in front of your partner; she may be nauseated by the smell or reminded that she should not have it.
- **Illicit drugs or prescribed drugs not as prescribed but to cope**: Few coping mechanisms have the formidable dissociative effect of drugs. They change the way we feel, perceive, and respond to everything. Finding yourself will be impossible when you are not yourself.
- **Aggression**: in words, actions, and reactions. Negative reactive behaviour includes more than only physicality. Subtle aggressions like impatience, gritting teeth, disapproving looks, and angry voices carry the same trauma and negative impact as their physical counterparts. Unless you address this, they will be impossible to stop. This is also a behaviour that will have a complex effect on a developing persona.
- **Rationalization**: If you find yourself reacting in a self-justifying manner to any of these points, try to be honest with yourself and

ask yourself, "Why?" Why would you try to defend something you know is not good for you unless the attachment to it is inappropriate?

Quitting or minimizing these habits will support your partner's health and yours. She wants to live clean, eat well, and exercise for the health of your baby, and she needs your help. You have to be a catalyst for the change and a companion on the journey, not a stumbling block.

Remember this is not about denying yourself things; this is about raising your self-awareness around what they do for you and to you. You should also ask yourself if they are behaviours you would like to pass on to your child. If you choose to do something, be honest with yourself about it so you can accept it as part of what you currently need to do. Then it becomes a matter of looking at how you can incorporate it into your life with a minimum of harm to those you love and yourself. This self-honesty and positivity will allow you to grow in other areas, leading to greater personal fulfillment, happiness, and ultimately termination of the negative behaviour.

You will also become accustomed to being a role model for your future child. Even more importantly, living healthy will help ensure that you are there to be the father your child needs. Now is the time for both of you (if you haven't started already) to begin your active lifestyle.

Take Stock of Yourself

Your wife isn't the only parent who needs to see the doctor. Make an appointment to get yourself checked out with your regular doctor. Let the doctor know that you are embarking on a change for the better and you want the "once over." Ask to have your weight, cholesterol levels, and blood pressure checked. When you go back for your next checkup, you can amaze your doctor with the improvements you have made through the Adrenaline Factor.

Expect Changes in the Bedroom

Be prepared for ups and downs when it comes to interest in sex from your partner. She is going through a lot of changes physically and emotionally, and both of those aspects have huge effects on each other, creating even more uncertainty. So the best thing for you to do is remain supportive (no whining). Don't worry, this won't always be the case. In the meantime, you can always give the palm sisters a call.

Maintain your attention with your partner; do not let yourself get distracted by your hectic daily life and miss what is going on with her and her body. At some point, she will start feeling her body's magic and look at you with loving eyes. Romance will be the word of the day. Let her know that you notice and tell her how attractive she is to you. Her pregnant glow and the filling out in all the right places is a temporary bonus—take advantage of it while you can.

Every man has concerns when it comes to sex with his pregnant partner and understandably so; there's a baby in there now. The best way to deal with this is to talk about it. Many people are not used to talking about sex but that's okay. It's okay to feel a little awkward talking about sex and it's okay to not feel awkward at all; we are all different. Start simple, keep the conversations upbeat, and have a smile on your face. Find out what is comfortable for her and talk about concerns you both may have. Establish your comfort zones so you can both relax and be honest. Remember you can also ask your doctor. They've heard it all before, so there's no need to be embarrassed. Get your questions answered and then you don't need to worry.

Survive Her Hormones

The hormonal changes going on inside your loved one are nothing short of miraculous. She is actually creating another human being inside of her—a little one who is part of her and you. The physiological rollercoaster rumbling through her body is extreme and highly demanding in every capacity. It is also what her body needs to do, to do the job properly.

She may react more strongly or differently than usual. She may cry at television ads or go ballistic over the wrong brand of milk. A simple event can be catastrophic, making her mind race. For example, she may have a moment like, "Where's my toothbrush? I can't even look after a toothbrush, how am I going to look after a child? I'm going to be the worst mother in the world!" As hard as it may be, try not to get caught up in the emotion of the situation. You are there to be her anchor, her comfort, and her link back to the here and now (*aka* reality).

Remember not to try too hard to "fix it"; it's more important that you are there to connect with her, to be there to hear her. As you remind her of where she is and how well she is doing, remind yourself you are doing your part. Sometimes we all just need to have a "moment" and your pregnant partner automatically qualifies for the extended patience program. You are creating a safe and supportive environment for you, your partner, and your child.

Miscarriage

Miscarriage is most common in the first three months of pregnancy, which is why many doctors suggest waiting past the three-month period before sharing your exciting news. Many women spontaneously miscarry their first pregnancy in this trimester. If she does miscarry, make sure you are on point: stay alert and available to console and comfort her, and encourage communication. Refrain from "should have" comments or having an opinion. It is important to make sure she continues to nourish and care for herself, as she may also be dealing with nausea, bleeding, and discharge. These of course will have a very different impact, making the experience quite different for her. Even if it's early in the pregnancy, a miscarriage is a real loss. Friends and family will want to console you, but can say the wrong thing. Remember that they mean well—they just don't know what to say.

Be sure to also allow yourself and your partner time to grieve and acknowledge the loss. Recognize your emotions without going into negativity. As it is early in the pregnancy, you may not be sure what to feel and you may be questioning why you are not more upset.

There is no "right" way to feel. Be authentic and come from your truth and that will be the correct way for you (always, in all things). Miscarriage is nature telling you something was not right with the process. Don't make it personal or torture yourselves looking for a reason or something (especially not *someone*) to blame.

When the time is right, if you choose to, allow yourself to learn what you can about the event and move forward together.

What You May Be Feeling during the First Trimester

You will find yourself going around almost as if you are a bit unhinged yourself. It's an odd thing: although you are not going through any of the physical and physiological changes your partner is, you will find yourself crying at the drop of a hat. A song on the radio or watching a movie about love and families (or actually pretty much anything at this point) might get you that indoor pool you always wanted.

Where you thought you were a typical man regarding your emotions or your ability to control them, fatherhood is here to dispel that belief. This is a good time for you to consider your definition of strength. Perhaps you are of the mind, as I was, that being a typical man consists of being a tough guy, disciplined, inflexible, and unaffected. Boy, was I wrong. These are all fear- and denial-based states that are necessary to maintain a fear-based, superficial lifestyle. These types of perspectives are also necessary to have if you are not based in your truth, living by uncertain knowledge in a fragile reality.

True strength comes with patience, kindness, and acceptance. I am not saying we men are to be doormats; quite the contrary. With these strengths also come knowledge, peace, and balance through which we will know when it is appropriate to maintain and protect our boundaries for ourselves and our loved ones.

Be a Man—Love

Our emotions are an integral part of this beautiful ride in becoming a father.

Do not despair—if you think this will go away, it won't. It only gets worse (or better depending on how you decide to look at it).

Know that it is okay to feel, and that through acknowledging your feelings, you honour yourself and provide the opportunity to process the emotion, to gain awareness, and to grow from the experience. Doing so will increase your confidence and strength; you will gain a better knowledge and understanding of yourself. This will allow you to be able to understand and support your loved ones, rather than reacting and trying to "fix" things.

Emotions let us know what is going on both in us and around us. When we don't acknowledge emotions, we don't deal with them. Think of the experience as a brick and the emotion surrounding the experience as a bubble floating inside us around the brick. When we acknowledge the emotion, we allow it to process and the bubble pops. The brick falls down and becomes part of our foundation making us stronger. When we do not acknowledge an emotion, the bubble remains with the experience, still active around it and inside of us. Similar experiences will activate and link with the initial experience and emotion. Soon you will have a bunch of bricks in a really big bubble; that's an extra load no one needs, a load you will keep trying to pretend is not there creating inner conflict and stress.

Unheeded emotions will manifest as something else, like anger, frustration, depression, and anxiety or a physical problem like illness or injury.

Right now, you may be feeling a bit unappreciated, unattractive, or even inadequate. These are feelings which—when added to the new challenges that come with pregnancy—can shake even the most confident man. Try not to let these feelings occupy too much time or space in your head, turning them to worry. Be sure to acknowledge and accept them as being how you feel and ask yourself where they may be coming from and why. As you allow yourself to work through them (feel them), you will be able to identify the original experience that gave the unease its beginning, providing opportunity for the unresolved emotion from the past to work through, popping the bubble, growing and healing in the process.

Share your feelings with your partner, though first check in with your truth around your motivation for doing so. Do not let that negative voice come in through expectations (do not have any; she is not a mind reader).

The game plan for this first trimester is being supportive, positive, and open. Listen to her hopes and fears, share her excitement, and get used to rolling with what life throws at you!

Bonus Tip #1
Do not look at other women.

Super Bonus Tip #2
Do not look at other women.

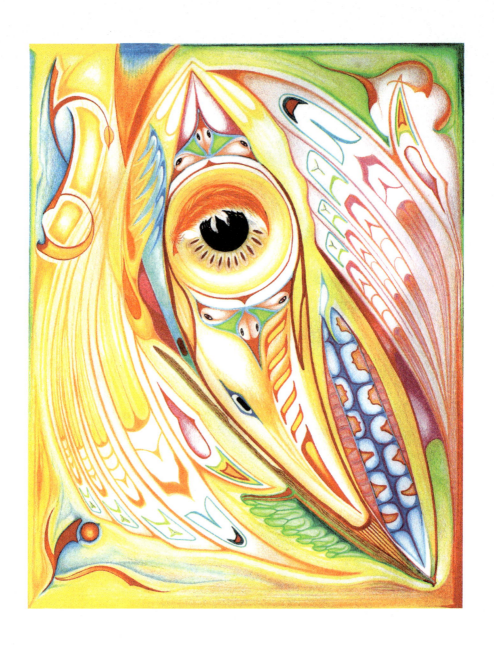

Second Trimester

Chapter 5 The Three Main Food Categories

Protein—The Building Block

Protein is important because it is the building block of our bodies, from our bones to our hair. It's involved in functions both inside and outside our cells, throughout our body's various systems and functions. Protein is essential to the repair of muscles after a workout.

With the Adrenaline Factor, your protein comes from what you may have heard referred to as "clean" food; this just means natural—sources that are low in fat and low in saturated fats. Let's just call it "real food." Either we killed it or picked it, straight from nature to your mouth.

"Clean" also refers to unprocessed. That means it has not been manipulated or altered in any way from its natural form and nothing has been added: no additives, preservatives, colours, or anything you have a hard time pronouncing. The ingredients list should be very simple. For example, the ingredients on a box of chicken breasts should say "chicken breasts" and not include a list of additives like soy protein, modified corn starch, salt, or water, to name a few. Water may sound harmless (which it is), but why would they be adding it to chicken? Water is heavy, so they can sell us less chicken for the same price. Water can carry additives, which do various things like add flavour and colour.

You may also be wondering how much protein to eat in a day. This is a good question and you will find opinions that range from 0.7 grams per pound of your body weight (0.7 g/lb.), to 2 g/lb. I recommend around 1 g/lb. a day. So if you weigh 175 pounds, you'd want around 175 g of protein per day, especially if you are going to be active and getting your muscles working.

The reason I say "around" 1 g/lb. is because eating does not need to be an exact science and I don't want you to get caught up in the numbers. Everyone is different and you need to find out what works for you; 1 g/lb daily is a good starting point. I would recommend if in doubt to err on the higher side. Protein is a good thing and will help your body recover and find its balance both metabolically (digestion and cellular function) and hormonally (emotion, energy, and recovery).

The recommended daily allowance (RDA) of protein in America and Canada is 0.8 g/kg of body weight (approx. 0.32 g/lb.). With an increase in activity, you will require more than the RDA in my opinion, as we need to add protein to compensate for the increased demand in energy maintenance and tissue repair.

I would like you to view food preparation with self-care and creativity, not as something that is all about the numbers and "things I can't eat."

If you are doing the workouts and find you are feeling tired or your muscles are sore for more than three days, you may not be getting enough protein. You can try increasing your protein intake by a few grams each meal.

Great clean sources of protein

- Chicken or turkey breast
- Fish, such as sole, cod, haddock, salmon, trout, sardines, and tuna
- Egg whites
- Beans
- Greek yogurt and tzatziki

- Nuts
- Lentils

Carbohydrates—The Fuel

Carbohydrates are a very important category; they are also frequently the scapegoat for our dieting woes. The main reason they carry this stigma is because they are yummy. We have a tendency to eat a lot of them, especially in Western society. And the majority of the time, they are processed or refined in some way.

All carbohydrates are basically sugar, converted from whatever they started as to glucose or blood sugar; glucose is the preferred source of energy for our bodies. Carbohydrates are also used for cellular function in our body and especially our brain. The glucose is converted to glycogen in our muscles and is what powers us through our resistance workouts.

Muscle glycogen is used up during our workouts, so post workout is a good time to have carbohydrates, either simple or complex. Pair your carbs with a protein to maximize glycogen-storage replenishment (fuel) and protein synthesis (muscle repair).

There are three different kinds of carbs: simple carbohydrates or sugars; fibrous carbohydrates; and complex carbohydrates.

Simple Carbohydrates or Sugars

The sweet stuff can be found in things like candy, syrup, fruit, juice, and milk. Figure out how you respond to sugar and try to have it around your workouts if you need to. It is absorbed very quickly by the body for energy, but has little to no nutritional value. Limit your intake of sugar; keep it to natural sources (no added sugar). This will not be as easy as it sounds. It may be called a simple carbohydrate, but identifying it can be quite complex. Companies have manipulated sugar for a multitude of reasons, one being to make it less identifiable.

Some of Sugar's Aliases

Here is a list of some of sugar's aliases: agave nectar, barley malt, barley malt syrup, beet sugar, brown rice syrup, brown sugar, buttered syrup, cane juice, cane juice crystals, cane juice solids, cane sugar, caramel, carob syrup, coconut palm sugar, coconut sugar, corn sweetener, corn syrup, corn syrup solids, date sugar, dehydrated cane juice, dehydrated fruit juice, dextran, dextrin, dextrose, diatase, diatastic malt, ethyl maltol, evaporated cane juice, fructose, fruit juice, fruit juice concentrate, fruit juice crystals, glucose, golden syrup, high-fructose corn syrup, honey, invert sugar, lactose, malt syrup, maltodextrin, maltose, palm sugar, raw sugar, refiner's syrup, rice syrup, saccharose, sorghum syrup, sucrose, syrup, treacle, turbinado, turbinado sugar, xylose, and anything ending in "ose."

I know; right! Don't worry. You may be thinking, "Am I supposed to memorize all these sugar aliases now!" The answer is no. I have included this (albeit incomplete) list of names to illustrate how confusing and seemingly complex the food industry makes the task of eating well. They will even put multiple types of sugar in a product in order to bury it further down the ingredients list, so it is not so obvious how much sugar is actually in the product. We will cover how to combat this with reading the nutritional information on labels later on.

This is another excellent reason to keep it simple and keep it about real food; then you do not need to worry about any of that food industry nonsense.

Fibrous Carbohydrates

Fibrous carbs come from vegetables. Fibre does not come from animal sources. Vegetables are full of micronutrients and their fibre keeps our digestive tract clean. Low in calories and high in nutrients, vegetables are an excellent choice anytime. Some veggies even have a negative caloric value: it takes more energy to eat and metabolize them than the calories they contain. Celery is an example of this (unless you make a Cheez Whiz boat out of it).

Complex Carbohydrates

These are found in foods like whole grains, whole grain pasta, starchy vegetables, peas, and beans. These are naturally nutritionally rich and satiating (helping us feel like we have had enough). Unfortunately, the food industry has manipulated our gifts from nature into enticingly marketed, colourfully boxed, emotion-numbing cash cows. These are the refined carbohydrates that act just like simple sugar. I felt it was necessary to look at these a little closer to better understand the complexity and depth of what we are facing.

Whole Food (Whole Grain)

Now is the time I would like you to pay close attention—if you take nothing but this point from this book, it will make a difference in your life forever. It most certainly has in mine.

Every carb you eat should be a whole food; your rice, grains, fruit (not fruit juice), and vegetables. The reason I put "Whole Grain" in brackets is because of the word games the food companies and their marketing campaigns like to play. A good example of this is the term "whole wheat." In Canada, marketers can sell a product as "whole wheat" if it has up to 70% of the germ missing; whereas "whole grain" must constitute 100% of the grain's different parts.

A whole grain is not only more nutritionally dense, but the body knows what to do with it; it is what nature has intended. It will feed your body longer and leave you more satiated.

Let's take a look at white flour. When ingested, white flour is very quickly absorbed by the body because all the nutrients and fibre—the dense or "brown" parts—have been removed. The reason for this is so the flour can sit on a shelf and not go bad. Yes, that's right. Even mould has more sense than we have.

White flour causes the body's sugar level to shoot up, rather than being slowly increased as would be the case with whole grain, and the body (pancreas) oversecretes insulin just like it would with processed or junk food. Insulin regulates (stores) carbohydrates and other nutrients such as protein in your body, shuttling them around. The insulin will carry glucose to the muscles for our glycogen stores. Unfortunately, there is a limited amount of glycogen storage in the muscles. Again, we have a large amount of sugar in the blood stream (from carbs), an abundance of insulin being released. The limited amount of room for glycogen storage in our muscles leaves sadly only one option: the insulin will take the remainder and store it as fat for which there are unfortunately no limits.

This is the rollercoaster ride your body goes on every time you eat something processed. That tuna salad on white you had for lunch is one of the worst things you could eat. Not only was the white bread like straight sugar, but the mayo in the tuna sandwich is straight fat (more on fats shortly), which with the increased insulin level from the white bread is easily stored as fat.

These fast-digesting sugar and other insulin-spiking foods are called high GI foods (Glycemic Index). I like the graph below because it illustrates the "crash" you get after the body has done its job. To cope with the abnormally high sugar level, your body releases an abnormally high amount of insulin, taking the sugar from the blood. There is a rebound effect—a low blood sugar state that significantly affects your levels of energy, cognitive (brain) function, and mood.

If this sounds a lot like the high and then the withdrawal of drugs that's because it is.

… Exactly the same

Professor Bart Hoebel and his team in the Department of Psychology at the Princeton Neuroscience Institute have been studying signs of sugar addiction in rats for years. Until now, the rats under study have met two of the three elements of addiction. They have demonstrated a behavioural pattern of increased intake and then shown signs of withdrawal. His current experiments captured craving and relapse to complete the picture.

Hoebel has shown that rats eating large amounts of sugar when hungry, a phenomenon he describes as sugar-bingeing, undergo neurochemical changes in the brain that appear to mimic those produced by substances that get abused, including cocaine, morphine, and nicotine. Sugar induces behavioural changes, too. "In certain models, sugar-bingeing causes long-lasting effects in the brain and increases the inclination to take other drugs of abuse, such as alcohol," Hoebel said ("Sugar can be addictive, Princeton scientist says" by Kitta MacPherson. *Princeton University News*, December 10, 2008).

Hoebel and his team also found that a region of the brain known as the nucleus accumbens releases a chemical known as dopamine when hungry rats drink a sugar solution. Dopamine is thought to trigger motivation and, eventually with repetition, addiction.

Foods high in sugar and processed foods will give us the "sugar binge" mentioned here coupled with dopamine release and followed by withdrawal. This is illustrated by the "High GI" graph below.

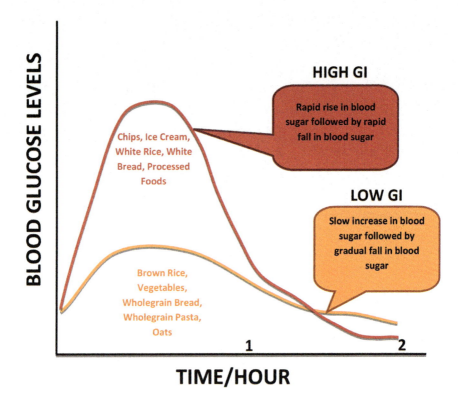

Fats

What's Wrong with Fat?
Answer: NOTHING.

We need fat to survive. Fats are essential for energy, metabolism, protection, organ and bone development, cognitive function, and hormone production. Some of the vitamins we need are fat soluble, which means we can use them only when they are combined with certain fats. Fats are the third member of our three macronutrient food groups.

Good and Bad Fats

Some healthy fats are the unsaturated Omega 3, Omega 6, and Omega 9 fats. Omega 3 fat can be found in salmon, sardines, and flaxseed oil; Omega 6 is in avocado, almonds, and peanuts (peanut butter); and Omega 9 is in avocado, olive oil, and macadamia oil.

The good fats actually help reduce LDL (low density lipoprotein) and increase the level of HDL (high density lipoprotein) in our bloodstream. This helps keep our arteries clear and everything flowing easily. The LDL (low density) means they are light and prone to piling up, clogging the arteries.

Be on the lookout for saturated fats and keep them to a moderate level. Saturated fats are necessary for things like testosterone production but also are the kind that increase your LDL and block up your arteries. These are also the fats that increase subcutaneous fat (the fat under our skin that makes us look fat), which especially for men in the abdominal area is linked to a higher risk of cardiovascular disease. Keep your saturated-fat intake from whole (real) foods and in moderation, and you will be okay. They can be found in dairy products like cheese and cream and also in the white fat in red meat, pork, and chicken.

Read the Nutritional Information on everything you buy. It will tell you how much saturated fat is there. Be mindful of the percentage per serving. Most foods that are high in fat are low in fibre, fibre being what helps us feel full and limits how much we eat. If you can eat your fats without carbohydrates, that is ideal. So carbs during the day when you are active and fats in the evening is a structure that works for me. A starting point for fats can be 0.3-0.4 g/lb. of body weight, which works out to 60-80 g of fat for the day for a 200 lb. person.

Unhealthy fats, or fats to avoid, are hydrogenated fats and partially hydrogenated fats and oils.

Trans fats deserve a section all their own. Though these occur naturally in red meat and some dairy products, the main source of these is from food that is packaged as "food products": most snack food and fast food. Trans fats in packaged food increase the LDL and decrease the HDL; the exact opposite of what we want. If you had a stick of butter in front of you or a stick of margarine, the right choice would be the butter. Margarine is a man-made evil that was initially full of trans fats and a laundry list of chemicals. Many still are, though they try to add oils like olive oil to enable marketing them as healthy.

The Risks of Consuming Too Much Fat

Fat contains twice as much energy (calories) as our other macronutrients, so there's a greater potential for it not to be fully used as fuel, and the excess stored as body fat. Excess body fat clogs up blood vessels and arteries, increases the risk for diabetes, high blood pressure, stroke, heart attack, negative self-image, low energy, and emotional issues to name a few.

Fat also makes us larger, which causes stress on our back and joints. It has been estimated that for every 22 lbs. of extra body fat there are 18 miles of extra blood vessels. That's extra mileage you absolutely do not need and a huge additional load for your heart.

7 Easy Ways to Eat Less Fat

1. Use skim milk instead of 2% or homogenized and nonfat Greek yogurt instead of sour cream.
2. Use nut butters and other spreads like light cream cheese or no-sugar jams sparingly. Use half of what you use now.
3. Grill, steam, poach, or bake your food.
4. If you use a frying pan don't pour oil into the pan. Coat it by rubbing the pan with an oiled cloth or use a non-stick spray. Better yet, use a nonstick pan with a little water instead of oil.

5. Trim the excess fat from pork and beef; remove the skin from poultry.
6. Use low-fat cheeses.
7. Eat a high protein and low GI carb for breakfast (egg whites and oats with a little cinnamon). This will start the day right and reduce late-night snacking.

7 Problems with Fat Free

1. Just because a prepared food is "fat-free" doesn't mean that it won't end up being stored as fat in your body. Many foods labeled "fat-free" are loaded with sugar, salt, and synthetic food substitutes like gums and flavouring.
2. Less fat usually translates to less flavour, so food manufacturers add more sugar, salt, and chemicals. These carbohydrates can be used as fuel, but once they have been used and the limited glycogen storage is reached, the excess goes into the blood stream and eventually the liver where it is converted to fat.
3. We need fat for proper hormone function, especially when we are increasing activity level.
4. Knowing we are eating low fat makes reaching for that extra helping a bit more justifiable; you may end up eating more because of that.
5. Eating "fat-free" may cause us to eat empty calories. For example, look at the difference in the calorie count between a "Fat Free" (and nutritionally void) pack of licorice (375 calories per 100 g) and a nutrient-rich boneless, skinless chicken breast (164 calories per 100 g).
6. Fat in food aids in providing a feeling of satiety, preventing us from overeating.
7. We can also become deficient in fatty acids. Physical signs can be dry skin, eczema, dry hair, soft or brittle nails. Other signs can

be problems with attention and concentration, and emotional issues like depression and anxiety.

Water

Drink 12 to 16 cups of water a day. These amounts are for everyone to start with. Optimal water consumption will help with everything from muscle fullness and skin health to bowel regularity. You might notice if you feel like having a snack that you may not have had any water for a while. Our signal for thirst often feels like hunger. So drink some water (one and a half to two cups) to help with the cravings. Drinking adequate amounts of water is a key component in promoting lean body mass (muscle) and reducing adipose accumulation (fat gain).

How to Start Applying This Information

Before the stress of "I am going on a diet" kicks in, I want you to understand that I am recommending that you eat more. Yes, I said "more." Diets and restrictions, tricks and quick tips are all marketing B.S. I want you to think "nourishment" for your mind, body, and soul. Food is our friend and is what keeps our bodies and minds going strong.

I am going to ask you to eat every two hours. That's right, every two hours. For example, if you are up at 7:00 a.m. to perform your morning workout, you will have breakfast by 8:00 and eat again at 10:00, 12:00, 2:00, 4:00, 6:00, and 8:00. Hopefully you will be going to bed by 10:00 p.m., although 9:30 would be better. Remember your partner is hard at work building a human, so she will be hungrier than pre-pregnancy, wanting to eat more often. This is a great opportunity for both of you to develop a regular two-hour eating structure with balanced nutrition together.

Eating early and often is important for getting the maximum

benefits from food. Our bodies are wonderful adapters, constantly seeking homeostasis (balance). When we wake up, our metabolism is looking to turn on and fire up. What we do in the morning will dictate the rest of the day, so breakfast is the most important meal. Our bodies have been fasting all night and we wake up in a stressed state; a good breakfast will turn your metabolism on with protein and keep you feeling full longer with a low GI carb, giving your brain some glucose to keep you sharp.

When you skip breakfast and don't eat until later, it's like putting your body into a double starvation mode. When this happens our metabolism and our energy level drops and any food that comes in will be divided up: some for work (energy and essential functions) and the majority for storage (fat) as your body prepares for the next fast. This is why you crave a high-calorie bang when you let yourself get hungry: your limbic system is hitting the panic button and wants a dump of calories to calm it down.

There are several reasons for eating every two hours

- You'll be eating real food—the kind your body knows what to do with, and loves to digest and metabolize. Because it's full of nutrients, your body will feel full and sated faster and give you the full signal earlier, meaning you'll eat less.
- You keep your body fed. No true hunger leads you to be able to identify cravings much more easily, by allowing you to ask yourself, "I just ate, so if my body is not hungry, what am I feeding?"
- Eating every two hours establishes a structure and an increased focus on self-care. This will aid in reducing mindless snacking when watching television or surfing the net, reducing overeating.
- Eating this way also keeps it simple to move in your desired direction, especially in the beginning of your journey when new routines are unfamiliar. When you are just starting to develop

a new schedule and routine, there's a danger of straying off course. Eating every two hours takes off some of the pressure, by providing a clear path of what and when to eat.

It will take two to three weeks for the new routine to find its rhythm. That will be the tough part, so keep it simple and don't give yourself opportunities to stray. This process will also aid you in "letting go." Letting go of your sense of control frees you from the stress of having to decide what, where, or how to eat.

Removing the burden of choice will make the beginning of your journey much easier. The brain knows what it wants and will manipulate our actions to get it. We must put some distance between the behaviours we are trying to change and the development of our new ones; we must allow ourselves to gain some clarity and resolve; and we must establish new behaviours (which will come with time) before introducing too many options.

Eating this way also prepares you for fatherhood, because babies and children usually need to eat every couple of hours. If everyone is on the same cycle, everyone eats at the same time, adding connection and peace to your routine.

Eating every two hours is optimal, but it can be difficult, especially in the beginning when you're still getting used to the new schedule. If you get delayed or forget, don't worry, just try to get reorganized within the hour—I don't want you going more than three hours between meals. We have been procrastinating our self-care long enough. It is time to break that behaviour pattern and step up. When we wait longer than three hours, our bodies start to go into starvation mode (just like skipping breakfast). Our metabolism slows down, and the systems being allocated energy (food) start to be selected on a priority basis. We lose our focus and start to become physically and cognitively effected (once you are hungry all bets are off). Then once you eat again, fuel storage as fat for future need starts to become more important than utilization (building and burning for recovery and energy).

Get used to making yourself and your nutrition a priority. Doing so will increase your balance and tranquility both mentally and physically, giving you the ability to effectively handle any challenge. Don't minimize yourself, your worth, or your potential. The martyr methodology is a popular one. Unfortunately, it is used as a grandiose rationalization: "I would die for my wife" or "I would die for my kids." That may be true and nothing to scoff at. That is something we default to when we feel perhaps less-than or question what we have of value to offer.

Build your foundation and find your truth. Begin to realize you are enough and always will be. Live by example: support and guide your family.

Don't die for them, LIVE for them.

How to create a strong foundation

You're probably saying, "That all sounds great but where do I start?"

You start by creating a clean slate for yourself. How we do that is by removing the poisons and creating a new foundation to work from. It can all be very confusing especially if you have some experience with diets, fasting, superfoods, gluten-free, etc. This is why we are starting bare bones and keeping it real easy: real food, that's it. Simple, focused, and progressive.

Complexity is the cave in which justification lurks.

Clear the Room

Let's start in the kitchen. Have a look at anything white in your cupboards—enriched flour, sugar, bread, rice, pasta, and cereal. Pack it up and either give it away or throw it away.

After studying the diet records of 2,300 people, Italian scientists concluded that eating more than four slices of white bread a day doubles a person's risk of developing kidney cancer. The white stuff is processed to give it a long shelf life and prevent mould (life). When these foods are refined (turned white), most of their nutrients are lost, greatly diminishing their health benefits and disease-fighting capabilities, not to mention significantly increasing the likelihood that they will be stored as fat.

In the grand scheme of things, white foods are not the worst bad guys, but they should at least be replaced by their brown counterparts.

STOP

I do not agree with the accommodating tone of this sentence—"white foods are not the worst bad guys"—but I left it in for a reason. When I initially wrote this section, that is how I started it. When reading it again later, the irresolution of the statement was much clearer to me. I draw my line at white flour, meaning I don't eat it, because it is one of the bad guys. So why would I say "white foods are not the worst bad guys"? That is exactly the type of rationalization I am trying to help you identify and change in yourself!

So what a great opportunity for me to ask myself, "Why be irresolute?" What I came up with is I felt uneasy because most people (sometimes, it feels like everybody) eat out and consume white flour, white rice, and white sugar. Heck, let's just say it. I was scared, scared of negative or conflictive feedback. I didn't want people saying or thinking, "He is just another health freak." In other words, my fear and false ego got in the way. To stand in our truth and go against custom, to stand alone against a majority are daunting propositions. Create the change within yourself. We don't need to convince anyone else when we lead the way with our actions.

Raising our awareness of these kinds of responses and processes as they happen within us is actively creating our foundations of change. Identifying what and how we react to circumstances, people, and things allows us to identify what we need to be curious about. It allows us to see how we get in our own way. We need to shine the light on and acknowledge what creates these mental, spiritual, physiological, and psychological responses.

When our friends (peers) and people around us (society) are acting in the same way, the external and internal pressure to conform or "go with the flow" is very intense; many built-in, subconscious processes are at work. I like to remind myself of the quote: "The opposite of courage is conformity." Stand strong in your truth. Before you can stand in your truth, you first need to figure out what your truth is. Be open and identify your reactions, but listen to the truth.

"People pretend not to like grapes when the vines are too high for them to reach," Marguerite de Navarre (1492-1549 AD).

Many sociobiological, physiological, and psychological factors are working without our conscious awareness. I list a few of them here so we can acknowledge the fact that it's not as simple as "making the right choice."

- Sociobiology theorizes that we have genes that aid group-survival behaviours. This means scientists believe we have genetic programming that influences us to go with the flow and be part of a group rather than go against it.
- Behaviour Genetics focuses on the influences of heredity and our individual traits and how we are more like those we are related to (reared by) than to other people (not related to or reared by).
- Evolutionary Theorists say we have predictive-adaptive responses. As we grow in the womb, we undergo genetic changes to give us the best chance of survival in our anticipated future environment.

- Neuroscience has given us the discovery of mirror neurons. These neurons in our brains are for imitation and emulation. They allow us to feel and/or experience (empathize) what others are doing, the same as if we were actually doing it ourselves.
- Physiological effects of endorphin release on the brain lead to the limbic system (subconscious brain) becoming highly motivated to seek out the stimulus, identifying what provides it, and telling the prefrontal cortex (conscious, working brain) how to get it. Conversely when the brain is activated by sugar/fat withdrawal (dopamine withdrawal), the increased cortisol levels from the stress associated create powerful craving and seeking impulses.
- Epigenetic factors can be linked to current influences such as our mother's or father's lifestyle, diet, and behaviours, and to past environmental influences of our ancestors. These variables influence gene activation and gene silencing, the turning on and off of genetic traits and behaviours, having a direct effect on everything from our actions to our metabolism.

Sprinkle all that with emotional coping, avoidance, add a scoop of being hungry, and your limbic system's survival instinct is about to override everything … you can put a cherry on that sucker because you have just created your own hot fudge sundae of "It's not about choice!" Great, now I feel like an ice cream sundae, even after saying all that!

If you are still reading, good. Acknowledgement is one of the hardest and most important steps. Identifying these aspects within yourself is great and gives us something to watch out for and to focus on, a place to start. We are not broken, not even close. We just need to figure out the behaviours and ideals we have been taught and assimilated that are working against us. Listen for the ugly voice; do not dismiss it or pretend it's not there; get to know it so you can recognize it when it speaks.

Chapter 5

**Know thine enemy for he is the architect of
your alibi and consort to your lethargy.**

This is all important. Have conviction and clarity in your knowledge. We must be secure and prepared in our truth, to keep our path simple and know what is good for us and what is not. So when we are tested, we can say, "No, thank you," without being reactive (not "Oh! How dare you offer me that!"). The reason I say "without being reactive" is because we want to be safe and at peace in our truth, without feeling like we need to explain or justify what we are doing and so we do not feel threatened or doubtful when someone scoffs or questions us. We also do not want to be judgmental. Lead by example not by preaching. That type of behaviour tends to come from people who are unsure or feeling threatened. A common coping mechanism is externalization (judgment/blame); it's common because it is so effective. It takes the focus off ourselves and directs it towards others, detaching us from what we are really feeling. Mind your own business and increase your self-awareness in the process.

When we see products in the stores, we want to assume they are safe and not a hazard to our health. We trust the "system"; well, the "system" is making us sick. The system currently in place is making money for the companies supplying it. Simply, it's a market economy not a wellness or health economy. One hundred percent whole grain bread, brown rice, whole GRAIN pasta, and whole grain cereal—real whole foods—are the only choices you should be making. Especially at the beginning of your new journey, you must keep it simple. I'm not saying all products are the devil; a few companies are trying to provide real food (they see the shift coming). Read the ingredients list. If a company is honestly trying to provide real food, then that's where the proof will be.

Learn to be patient with yourself and breathe. The ability to be patient with yourself will help your daily life, giving you the opportunity to be in the moment. You will hear your truth giving you the ability to direct and simplify your perspectives more clearly.

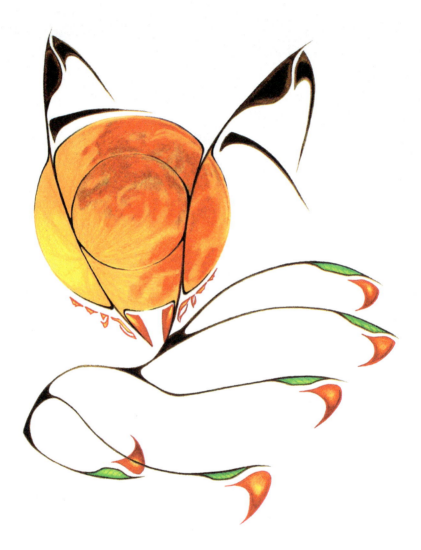

Chapter 6 The Phase 2 Workout

Welcome to Phase 2 of your Adrenaline Factor workout program! You should already be seeing and feeling positive changes, both physically and mentally. You will be experiencing improved energy levels, a positive outlook, and reduced stress. The simple self-care structure will accentuate balance in your life, helping you more easily identify those things not based in your best interest.

Now you have a basic biomechanical knowledge of how to move. You not only know how to move, but you know how it feels. They say knowledge is power; this is only true if that knowledge is applied. By doing the multi-joint exercises in the program, you will apply that knowledge, improving your skill, coordination, fitness level, and awareness in the process.

You have also made the transition from talker to doer.

We will now work on the mind-muscle connection. You will start to pinpoint specific areas of the body and which muscles are doing the work. This will allow you to make muscles stronger, more flexible and, if you desire, bigger. You will learn how to change the shape, structure, and capabilities of your body. You will gain the ability to focus on particular areas of it, to suit your fitness goals.

I am not talking about spot reduction. We often hear about magic fixes for love handles or are promised we will get a six pack by strapping an electro-shock stimulation pad or some new abs-slammer-jammer-twisty-springy gizmo to our belly. I want to make one point perfectly clear: there is no such thing as spot reduction when it comes to fat, unless you are talking about an invasive surgical procedure. Doing sit-ups will not give you a six-pack; you must reduce the subcutaneous adipose (fat) layer on top of them; period.

In Phase 2, we are using light weights and higher reps. We use the weights as tools to give the muscles resistance, which stimulates them to do what muscles were meant to do: work. We are not using our muscles to lift weights. The higher reps will give you the opportunity to better experience the "pump" in your muscles. This will really help you figure out which muscles are doing the work and enhance your mind-muscle (body) connection. I would also like to remind you that "weights" can mean anything from cans of beans to paper weights. You can also provide resistance for your muscles by flexing them as you move them through the movement. This is an excellent way to teach your body the exercise and enhance the connection between mind and body.

This is the time to check your ego at the door—not only do we have to accept our current capacity and ability, we also have to allow the experience to be new, and continue to build on the strong foundation we have already established. We also want to continue being curious as to how we move and how we can stimulate specific muscles in specific ways. Isolating the muscles will require less weight and an excellent opportunity to gain awareness of our egos. I have been doing this for thirty-five years and am thrilled to continue to make changes and new discoveries every workout.

The 30-rep range is designed for you to start feeling the burn at 15-20 reps, with the last 10 being more intense, keeping technique as the priority. If you reach muscular failure, stop the exercise. As you become more advanced, you can take a quick rest at muscular failure to let the lactic acid flush out of your muscles, then finish the rep count. This is a technique to increase the intensity of an exercise (again only after you have done a few weeks at Phase 2. Watch out for ego). DO NOT try to force the weight up.

If you need to rest more than twice before you reach the rep goal, you should lower the weight for your next set, especially during the first couple of weeks.

As your muscles begin to tire, your body will automatically begin to enlist other muscles and techniques (like swinging or jerking) to help you lift the weight. When you begin doing this, it means you have reached muscular failure for the targeted muscle group. Fight this natural tendency and stop. It is your job to maintain your form, which will increase the intensity, effectiveness, and efficiency of the exercise. Working out this way is actually much more productive than trying to force the weight up and you will experience less overall fatigue.

"Enjoyable lifting" is using weights that are appropriate; "stressful lifting" is trying to live up to your expectations.

Once you have established proper technique, your mental focus will be on the target muscle.

Monday

Target Muscle Group: Shoulders

15-Minute Morning Shot of Adrenaline

When: Before breakfast

Reps

12 forearm extensions on the ball on knees
12 side-to-side jumps holding arms out
6 per side: snatch press alternating sides
Perform as many sets as you can in 10 minutes. Rest as little as possible. Push yourself to go as fast as you can while maintaining proper form.

> **NEVER SACRIFICE PROPER FORM FOR SPEED OR WEIGHT! DO WHAT YOU CAN WHILE MAINTAINING PROPER FORM.**

20-Minute Body Sculpting

When: Anytime during the day

Reps

30 dumbbell military press seated on ball or chair
30 standing front shoulder raises
30 rear deltoid on ball or chair
Select a weight so you start to feel the burn at 20-25 reps. It will seem really light at first but keep the form STRICT! You can take a quick break at 20 reps to clear the lactic acid out of the muscle. Rest for 2-3 seconds but no longer.

Tuesday

> **Target Muscle Group: Legs**

15-Minute Morning Shot of Adrenaline

When: before breakfast

Reps

12 jumping jacks
8 step ups
12 ball punch crunches
Perform as many sets as you can in 10 minutes. Rest as little as possible. Push yourself to go as fast as you can while maintaining proper form.

20-Minute Body Sculpting

When: Anytime during the day

Reps

30 squats
30 straight leg deadlifts
30 jump squats
Select a weight so you start to feel the burn at 20-25 reps. It will seem really light at first but keep the form STRICT! You can take a quick break at 20 reps to clear the lactic acid out of the muscles. Rest for 2-3 seconds but no longer.

Wednesday

> **Target Muscle Group: Back**

15-Minute Morning Shot of Adrenaline

When: before breakfast

Reps

10 jumping jacks
10 push-ups
10 squat punches
Perform as many sets as you can in 10 minutes. Rest as little as possible. Push yourself to go as fast as you can while maintaining proper form.

20-Minute Body Sculpting

When: anytime during the day

Reps

30 dumbbell bent over row
30 towel row
30 one-arm ball rows
Select a weight so you start to feel the burn at 20-25 reps. It will seem really light at first but keep the form STRICT! You can take a quick break at 20 reps to clear the lactic acid out of the muscles. Rest for 2-3 seconds but no longer.

Thursday

Target Muscle Group: Chest

15-Minute Morning Shot of Adrenaline

When: before breakfast

Reps

12 ball punch crunches
12 side-to-side jumps on toes holding arms out
6 per side: snatch press alternating
Perform as many sets as you can in 10 minutes. Rest as little as possible. Push yourself to go as fast as you can while maintaining proper form.

20-Minute Body Sculpting

When: anytime during the day

Reps

30 chest press on ball or floor
30 chair dips
30 incline chest press on ball
Select a weight so you start to feel the burn at 20-25 reps. It will seem really light at first but keep the form STRICT! You can take a quick break at 20 reps to clear the lactic acid out of the muscles. Rest for 2-3 seconds but no longer.

Friday

Target Muscle Group: Arms

15-Minute Morning Shot of Adrenaline

When: before breakfast

Reps

12 forearm extensions on ball
12 side-to-side jumps on toes holding arms out
6 per side: snatch press alternating
Perform as many sets as you can in 10 minutes. Rest as little as possible. Push yourself to go as fast as you can while maintaining proper form.

20-Minute Body Sculpting

When: anytime during the day

Reps

30 biceps curls
30 triceps extensions on ball or floor
30 reverse grip biceps curls
Select a weight so you start to feel the burn at 20-25 reps. It will seem really light at first but keep the form STRICT! You can take a quick break at 20 reps to clear the lactic acid out of the muscle. Rest for 2-3 seconds but no longer.

Perception is learned.
Knowledge is earned.
Find your truth.

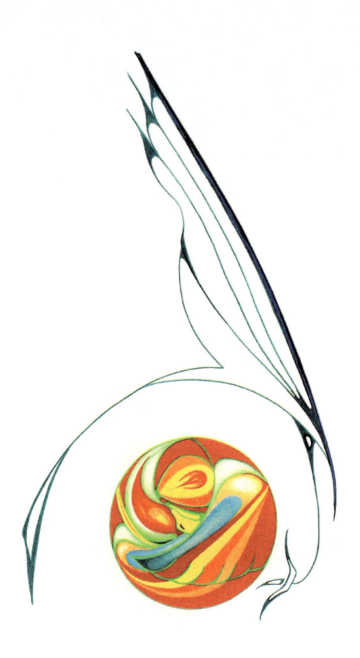

Chapter 7 Supporting Your Partner in the Second Trimester

What She's Experiencing: 8 Common Second Trimester Highlights

1. **Increased energy**: She'll get things done that she won't be able to do in the third trimester or after the baby's arrival.
2. **Improved mood**: Try and increase your communication; if you can do it now, it will help when times are more arduous.
3. **Increased sex drive**: Be open and available; if you think you are "getting the look," let her know you feel the same way.
4. **Improved self-image**: She will probably feel better about herself as she starts to look pregnant and may be enjoying a new maternity wardrobe.
5. **Having to pee all the time**: All the time.
6. **Decreased or no nausea**: Reactions to food, smells, and car travel may not be as severe, so some last nights out may be in order.
7. **Pregnancy glow**: Increased blood circulation will give her a healthy glow. She may experience certain areas of skin becoming darker, such as her face, nipples, and the line from her belly button to her pelvic bone. This is normal. If you decide to say something, keep it tactful and positive, but better yet avoid it.
8. **Preparing**: Her nesting instinct will be in full drive, so expect to use this time to make your home ready for the baby. Start

thinking about baby proofing your home and getting supplies such as a crib, change table, stroller, car seat, etc. (Friends and family may want to buy some or all of these for you. People love to give when you're starting a family. Learn to accept gifts and help graciously while being sure to maintain your boundaries.)

Things You Can Do to Strengthen Your Relationship and Your Role in the Pregnancy

Deal with the Physical Changes

During this trimester your partner will lose her waistline and start to gain a belly. You will see physical changes in her from a rounder face to bigger boobs. (I know I could have said "breasts," but "boobs" is way more fun. "Boooooooooooobs.")

She will enjoy looking obviously pregnant, but at the same time worry about how big she is getting. Although excited, she may also be feeling fat, tired, hungry, uncomfortable, or guilty after eating, fearful of labour and delivery, stressed from giving up her vices, and judgmental of herself when an attractive woman goes by (Remember Super Bonus Tip #2!). Remember that just because she may be feeling these things does not mean she wants you to know she is feeling them. Be discreet and supportive; never assume to know what she is going through, unless you want a well-deserved shot to the arm.

In her heightened emotional state, she may also feel that people are gossiping about her. This is your chance to be a source of strength and confidence for her. Step in and tell her that it doesn't matter what other people think and it's just that people like to share excitedly about seeing a pregnant woman. She is creating a human in there; oddly enough, people (humans) often relate to that.

Although she may seem to worry most about what other people think, who do you think she is most concerned about? You guessed it: You. She is worried about no longer being attractive to you. Give her compliments and not just words. Show her physically that she is still the apple of your eye. Go out of your way to let her know you think she's beautiful. Do not try to comfort her by reassuring her that everything will return to normal after the baby is born. A comment like that is laden with expectation, stress, and condemnation of her current state.

Do not falsely overdo it or say it in autopilot mode. The comments will very possibly have the opposite of their desired effect. You will also be denying yourself the warmth and peace that comes with giving an authentic loving comment. Positive honesty is the rule. We often think much more than we say; life is too short to let a loving thought go unrealized.

Bonus Tip #3

There is one exception to the positive honesty rule: there is only one answer to questions like "Do I look fat in this?" or "Is my bum saggy/too big?" and that is unequivocally "NO."

Absolutely under no circumstances are you to deviate or elaborate on this answer.

If she asks you to do so, immediately without hesitation light yourself on fire and run screaming from the room.

Stay Clear

As her physical appearance changes, she may worry about those changes being permanent. Looking in the mirror, she sees more of herself—a protruding belly, bigger bum, and puffier genitals. Even though these changes are temporary, she will be concerned about losing the weight and what her body will look like afterwards: will she have saggy breasts and stretch marks?

These are legitimate concerns, especially if you are brought up in a society where physical appearance and a materialistic value system are the norm. If her excess weight stays on, there can be negative physical and emotional effects, which may impact her wellness and possibly the stability of your family.

Truly these are the miracles of pregnancy and the amazing processes going on inside and outside your partner.

Stay present. Stay clear.

This will help you stay focused when worry creeps in. Put yourself in the present moment and do a quick check list. Check over your self-care: When did you eat last? When did you last have water? Where are you? Check in with your breathing, following it for 30 seconds.

Maintaining a regular schedule of self-care will give you the structure you need to stay present, creating for yourself and within yourself a place of positive energy and empowerment; you are not waiting for something to happen but creating outcomes.

The temporary part can be tricky but with you leading the way through healthy eating and exercise during the pregnancy, she will find it easier to regain her natural balance after pregnancy.

Eating properly is not only in the mother's best interest, but also that of her baby's. A developing fetus makes physical changes based on information and nutrition from its mother's body. The fetus tries to match its future environmental conditions. Teratogens are things that cause harm to the developing baby. In a developing fetus, neurons can grow at the rate of 250,000 a minute (4,167 new neurons per second). Vitamin deficiency, exposure to smoking, alcohol, and chemicals may damage or prevent neuronal development. The reason I bring up teratogens here is they are generally foreign agents to the natural processes that our bodies have evolved from and with. Things like processed foods and artificial flavours and colours (chemicals) are totally foreign and they can throw a wrench into the machine. If our weathered and beaten bodies do not know what to do with them, what effects will they have on a little developing fetus that has millions of cellular processes trying to create organs and tissues, turning on and off genetic codes, and trying to develop compatibility for the environment of its birth?

The mother's mental and emotional environment also has a major effect on the fetus and will also have an effect on which genes are activated in the child's development. This is one of the reasons a supportive, non-stressed environment is important for mom and baby.

Bonus Tip #4

She may be (more likely you are) over the moon about her bigger, fuller breasts. You can admire them but if you are asked, your answer will be, "I prefer your regular size" or "They were already perfect." If you feel otherwise, keep it to yourself—the change is only temporary but a self-centred comment is forever. Soon enough, they will go back to her pre-pregnancy size, a couple of pounds shy of regular pressure.

Be Decisive

No matter how excited and happy she is, your partner may be feeling a little overwhelmed right now. She may seem like she is handling things. In all probability, she wants you to help with making the decisions. Step up and take charge—now is the time to show her and yourself how ready you are to be a dad. Simple structure is a great way to minimize stress. Even if it's something as simple as "What's for dinner?", have the answer ready, and have a Plan B too. I am not saying take over; I am saying up your game so you are prepared to make decisions and stay involved in what's going on.

VIVA LA REVOLUTION!

The big bonus for you at this point is that along with a glowing partner with big firm breasts and heightened sensitivity in her genitals, she is having her own sexual revolution and wants nothing more than for you to be waving her flag.

Some men are too concerned with the pregnancy or not even thinking along those lines to catch the hints she may be dropping. Mark middle pregnancy on your calendar. As always, keep the lines of communication open so both of you can enjoy this unique period in time.

Remember that everything about her is more sensitive now, so a gentler touch may be best. Experiment with positions and make sure to ask her what is comfortable and what is too deep. A well-placed pillow may help, or a chair, or a countertop. Use the whole house while you still can—you will be relegated to closed-door bedroom sex soon enough.

Have a Last Hurrah

This is a time for you and your partner to do the things that you may not have time for with a baby. In this second trimester, she is not too big and may still enjoy most activities unencumbered. Middle pregnancy is usually the time when she has the most energy.

Sleep in, go on a spontaneous date, lie around naked, curse, and go out for dinner. This is also a good time to go on a trip, but if you do so, be your own advocate. If you plan on flying, check with your doctor first, and then check the weather forecast. Although the second trimester is the best time in the pregnancy for air travel, you still need to protect your family, and a bumpy ride may not be good for her or the baby.

Chapter 7

What You May Be Feeling during the Second Trimester

You may be feeling left out; don't. Expectations and lack of communication are often at the root of the misunderstandings and negative feelings we concoct in our minds. Your partner needs you and knows how important you are; that is all that matters. Don't wait to be invited, get involved—this is your baby too, so join in the planning and excitement. If it feels awkward or you don't know where to jump in, ask your partner and share some of your ideas and how you would like to get more involved. Being a father is so much more than the old stereotypes. Do not hold back. This is your time. You are going to be "Dad" now.

This is also a chance for you to grow. As your partner shows what she can do, show her what you can do. Lead by example. One of the ways you can do this is by applying the knowledge gained through the Adrenaline Factor and sharing it with her. After you have picked up some groceries and made lunch or dinner (making enough for the next day's meals also), discuss not only what you had but why you chose it and how it is better feeding your bodies and the baby's with clean, real food. Remember this is about increasing your awareness and being the change. With a new member of the pack on the way, you will have ample "justification" for being too busy and too tired.

Pregnant Dad Syndrome

Chances are that unless you have been following the Adrenaline Factor, you will be starting to show a few extra pounds too. "Sympathy pounds" is the common name for this and it is a real problem for men. That extra weight sneaks up on you slowly, and by the time you realize it, you, my friend, are deep (or deeper) in the hole.

It's natural for you to want to give her what she is craving and this can be a nice way to connect. To make her happy makes you happy. Food is a very common love language. Unfortunately, you are doing yourself and your partner a great disservice and creating a feedback loop that is very difficult to break. Unless, of course, you are following the guidelines from the Adrenaline Factor nutrition; then no worries—you're golden.

Going along with eating that quart of ice cream in front of the television will ease her guilt by sharing it, but the funny thing about eating crap is that the more you do it, the easier it becomes. When she starts to see your belly over the top of your pants or watches you huff and puff bringing in the groceries, she may blame herself or feel guilty for encouraging you to eat with her. I am not saying do not eat things like ice cream; just make the choices good ones, all natural, whole food, etc. Always remember to add a side of awareness with your snacks and of course, enjoy them guilt free.

Guilt (worry's nasty cousin) is an inhibitor of positive growth both physically and emotionally, and creates extra pressure that she doesn't need right now.

The truth is your condition, however it may be, is yours—taking ownership of that will always shift you from victim to empowered, giving you a place to stand and a place to start.

A largely unreported problem similar to sympathy pounds is "sympathy craziness." Your heightened emotional state and your close proximity to another heightened emotional state are the causes, but don't worry—you are not alone and this too will pass. Keep things simple and stick to the plan.

The Critic

As we have raised the topic of guilt, let's take a closer look. Say hello to the critic, the negative voice. It is the ugly little one inside of us that gets in the way of our potential. It supports negative self-perception and prevents us from taking positive risks.

The negative voice with its reactive emotions is established from a very early age and as we grow it grows with us, becoming a part of all our experiences from its inception. Unfortunately, it is very efficient at what it does and is applied to anything that resembles the primary experience. Ironically, it is initially established as a defense mechanism to protect us from pain experienced in the more challenging times of our lives. A guardian shouts at us, criticism, judgment, perceived failure, bullying; the list goes on and the pain is deep and personal. That initial pain is the birth of our critic created originally to prevent the same painful experience from happening again. Sadly, our protector becomes our prison.

This negativity wears many different hats. This is the innate creativity that all human beings possess, hard at work, regrettably in the wrong direction. We are using that creative energy to negate and minimize rather than to empower and maximize opportunity and experience in our lives.

Perhaps your boss gave you a hard time. You might be saying, "This is so unfair. I need a beer" or "He is a jerk." The externalization (blame) and noise the negative voice creates makes it easier for us to rationalize and consent to the contrived validity of our fear-based behaviours. When we are in a negative space with a negative perception, negative behaviour (self-harm and negative coping) fits very well.

Some examples of this perception are

- tough guy
- avoidance (distraction)
- judgment
- comparison
- anger
- control
- expectation
- denial
- blame

- defamatory humour
- minimization
- indifference

These will be well-practised behaviours that we accept as part of our personalities—the "way we are" or "who we are"—without giving them a second thought. The fact that these are subconscious responses makes them very difficult to catch.

The negative voice not only provides the perspective necessary to justify inappropriate coping mechanisms, it is a major player in creating the "issues" that distract you from noticing the harm and avoidance you are perpetrating upon yourself.

- "I'm not going to speak in the meeting, it's probably not a good idea anyway."
- "Sure I'm big; guys are supposed to have a little weight!"
- "Why should I worry? It's not like I'm going to play in the NFL!"
- "Everyone else is eating the donuts; I just had a half."
- "You have no idea of the pressure I'm under."

A bizarre part of this behaviour is we will set ourselves up with these types of statements to "prove" our point of view, manipulating the scenario for validation through a "See, I told you so" outcome. These types of statements based in half-truths, societally accepted norms and views are used to affirm negative self-perception. Somehow, the critic finds a way (albeit a very deleterious way) for us to feel validated through this negative feedback loop, which is why we need to keep it simple.

Subtlety is our critic's greatest weapon.

When emotion is triggered by a situation, the emotion rises, but because the defense mechanism is there to protect us from the pain of

Chapter 7

the emotion, the reaction is what comes out first.

Raising our awareness around these reactions will help us start to determine the true underlying emotion. When we acknowledge this we reveal our authentic self and gain access to our strength and potential.

Don't give away your power and let reactionary emotion blame everyone else. Rather, try to acknowledge your role and see the opportunity that has been created, the opportunity to become empowered to learn, to grow, and to change.

If you miss a day of exercise, or eat a dozen donuts, I honestly am not concerned, not in the slightest. I don't want you to be either. Try instead asking yourself, in an open, nonjudgmental way, "Why did I want to do something that is not good for me?" Chances are you won't know why, but that's okay. Allowing yourself not to know is not only the preferred but more dauntless answer, rather than filling the space with noise and complex justification.

Asking the question is the first step, allowing you to become present.

Endowing yourself with the gift of not knowing creates the space for wisdom.

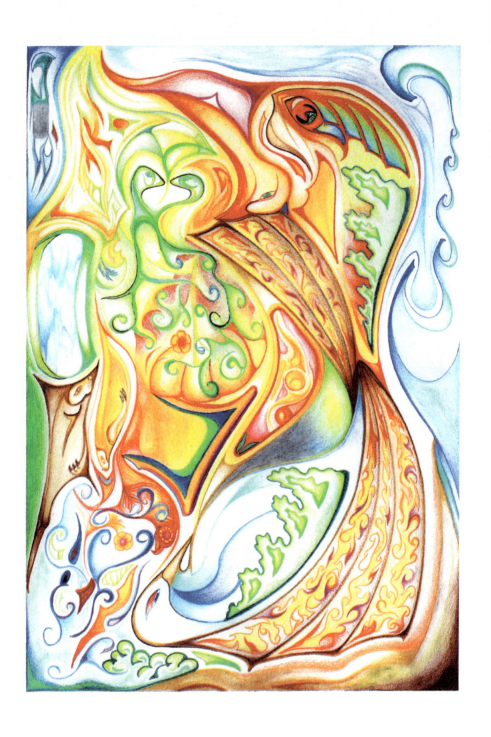

Third Trimester

Chapter 8 Eating Well—7 Rules for Success

1. Shop Weekly

It's best to eat fresh produce and fruit—locally grown and ripened if available. Keep an eye on specials for meat. This will help motivate you to look outside the normal routine and try something new. When you shop, get just enough veggies to cover your meals for the week including daytime snacks and watching-a-movie snacks. Be aware of what is in season as this produce will be the freshest and tastiest, and the prices will be lower also. Unfortunately, money is an issue for most of us; try to remember your priorities. Buy your socks on sale, not your food. If you need to make financial sacrifices do not make them with what you put in your body.

2. Make a Plan and Stick to It

Always have a list when you buy groceries. Make out your list before you set foot in the store. I recommend not buying anything that's not on the list, but if you do, it's a great opportunity to gain awareness about what the lure was that you were feeling. Remember this is about awareness. Awareness is not just about recognizing the desire to purchase something we know is not good for us but awareness is also about recognizing the guilt and shame we also feel after we have done so or after we have eaten it. Try to stick to the list though. Get in and out. This will help especially in the beginning of your journey to keep it simple until things start to make sense a little.

The other secret to success is to eat before you go grocery shopping. DO NOT GROCERY SHOP HUNGRY! Shopping when you're hungry almost guarantees you'll end up with some kind of processed convenience food. If you do get caught shopping hungry, you have two choices. First you can stop at the deli. Get a roasted chicken or something else that is real food—like whole grain bread, naturally cured meat, tzatziki dip for the chicken, low fat cheese, and pickles with whole grain crackers. Grab some veggies like broccoli or cauliflower or some fruit like apples and bananas. Buy them right away (anything sold by weight), start eating what you bought, and head back in to do your shopping as you check off your list. Your second choice is to find an individually wrapped item and eat it while you shop. Just remember to take the wrapper to the cashier to pay for it along with everything else. You are at a grocery store and there are lots of good options. Just don't fall for the traps. Have an idea of what you are going to get to eat before you go in and get it straight away.

At the grocery store, start on the outside aisles, where you find essentials like fruit and vegetables, skim milk, eggs, egg whites, whole grain breads and cereals, fish and meat. Stay out of the middle sections—they're usually full of snacks and processed, easy-to-prepare foods that generally have lower nutritional value, much higher calories, alluring packaging, and higher prices. Stay strong. Millions of dollars have been spent on product placement and packaging design to make you want to buy those items. Remember, don't buy a thing that's not on the list.

I would like to extend the "do not grocery shop hungry" to shopping in general. This is just as important and just as relevant. When you are at the mall, before you know it, a couple of hours fly by and you are hungry and without a meal. The next thing you know, you are standing in the food fair eyeing up Chinese fast food or some fries and gravy.

Ya, you know what I'm talking about. So take precautions to protect yourself from the sirens' song of the food court; you are only human after all.

3. Knowledge Is Power—Read the (back) Label!

Don't rely on anything on the label except the nutritional information and the ingredients list. Ignore the other parts of the label; they are the domain of the marketing experts. These people devote their professional lives to studying colours, shapes, layouts, and wordplay to manipulate you into buying the product they want you to, even if you don't. Words and phrases like "natural," "part of a healthy breakfast," or "home-style" can legally be used to misrepresent food, to make it seem healthier than it really is. "Low fat" and "reduced sodium" usually mean more sugar. The packaging is the hook designed to make a product stand out and make you buy one product over the competitors'. Watch out for the colour on the label. Lately a lot of food products have been changing the colour of their packaging. The colours have been changing to shades of brown, beige, and green to make a connection to the "natural ingredients, whole grain, and ecofriendly" movement. If there is a catch phrase that is popular or has been in the media, companies will use it to sell their product. "Gluten free" is a popular one these days. Remember gluten free often means rice flour—that is white (refined) rice flour—which is the same as white (refined) wheat flour, which is the same as (refined) sugar *aka* crap. Because you are trying to be more aware of what you are eating, you will be more likely to choose foods presented as being healthier; they may not be. Be watchful and look further. A Caesar salad will have as much fat as a side of fries.

Also be aware of the wording. "Made with" and "Made from" can mean entirely different things. A food may be "made with" 100% whole grain, but it's possible that only a little bit is 100% whole grain, and the rest is enriched flour (white flour) or some other processed flour or fillers. "Multigrain breads" are a good example of this. They may have a multitude of whole grains in them, but the first thing on the ingredients list is usually wheat flour.

It's now mandatory for food manufacturers to include the nutritional information of their product on the packaging and, as I said, this and the ingredients list is the only part of the label that counts. The following diagram shows what it will look like in most cases. Let me give you a few tips on how to read and make sense of it quickly.

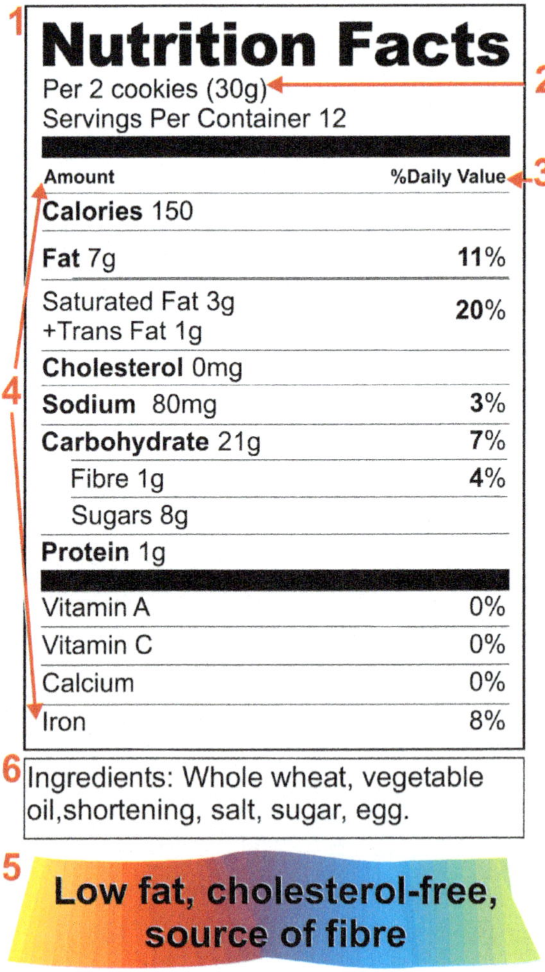

Nutrition Facts

Per 2 cookies (30g)
Servings Per Container 12

Amount	%Daily Value
Calories 150	
Fat 7g	11%
Saturated Fat 3g +Trans Fat 1g	20%
Cholesterol 0mg	
Sodium 80mg	3%
Carbohydrate 21g	7%
Fibre 1g	4%
Sugars 8g	
Protein 1g	
Vitamin A	0%
Vitamin C	0%
Calcium	0%
Iron	8%

Ingredients: Whole wheat, vegetable oil, shortening, salt, sugar, egg.

Low fat, cholesterol-free, source of fibre

1. **Nutrition Facts**: The listing of the main macronutrients and micronutrients.
2. **Serving Size**: Be sure the serving size is realistic—would you really eat only 4 crackers of this product or is it more likely to be 14? You can also use this guide to monitor your servings of this food and your total intake for the meal or snack to help figure your daily totals. Don't assume because it is individually wrapped that it is a single serving. Double check. I did that with a "protein brownie." I thought I read the nutrition facts (I saw what I wanted to see). I thought, "This is almost too good to be true." Well, it was. A serving was half a package (half a brownie). I was less than impressed. Who eats half a brownie! It was only midday and my carbs and fats were done for the day.
3. **Percent (%) of Daily Value**: This is useful if you are trying to raise or lower your intake of something like salt (sodium) or increase your level of vitamin C. Stick to the grams per serving ratio on the other items like fat, fibre, and protein for a more accurate per-meal check.
4. **Core Nutrients**: These are always listed in the same order for quick reference and comparison. Compare the amount per serving to the serving size. In this example, 3 g of a 20 g serving are fat. The big three are fat, carbohydrates, and protein. We want saturated fat to stay as low as possible. Do not consume anything that has "trans fats"—it's a red flag; VERY bad for heart health. We also want to be aware of the carbohydrate number unless we are talking about high-in-fibre carbs, which are great. Especially be mindful of high-in-sugar carbs, checking with the ingredients list for the sources of sugar. Protein is our friend. Get it however you can, the more the better.
5. **Nutrition Claims**: You can use these claims as a starting point, but use the nutritional facts and list of ingredients to make your final judgments.

6. **List of Ingredients**: The ingredients are listed in order of volume; if sugar is the first ingredient, then the product has more sugar in it than any other single ingredient. Use this to look for ingredients you wish to avoid. Sugar has many faces. I have provided some of its other aliases in chapter 4 to help you recognize your adversary's (the food industry's) devious ways: for instance, corn syrup, dextrose, fructose, glucose, malt syrup, invert sugar, and concentrated fruit juice. Look for an excess of chemicals and fillers. A good rule of thumb is the ingredients list should be small—the shorter the better. If there are things on the list you don't recognize, don't buy or eat the food.

Empower yourself by creating your safe space especially with what goes into your body. If you stay within your boundaries here, you will start more easily to identify the rationalization that subconsciously holds you back in the other aspects of your life. If you really want to eat something, make it yourself or find a substitute. I have come across food items I wanted to buy and I was hopeful they were healthy, due to clever naming like "whole wheat filo pastry" for example. Then I checked the ingredients list and yes, there was "whole wheat" but "wheat flour" was next on the list. Rather than justify the purchase, I allowed my frustration to be focused against those who are trying to trick us with their half measures, smoke-and-mirrors routine, attempting to capitalize on the false glimmer of hope they create with their lies.

They know the harm these items do (it's their business); yet they continue to prey upon the vulnerable amongst us and the vulnerabilities within us.

Comparing Cookies

Now that you're a label-reading expert, I'm going to give you a test.

Which of these cookies would you buy based on the nutritional facts? At first glance, they seem similar, but we're expert label readers now, so let's look deeper.

Label A

Nutrition Facts
Per 2 cookies (30g)
Servings Per Container 12

Amount	%Daily Value
Calories 150	
Fat 7g	11%
Saturated Fat 3g +Trans Fat 1g	20%
Cholesterol 0mg	
Sodium 80mg	3%
Carbohydrate 21g	7%
Fibre 1g	4%
Sugars 8g	
Protein 1g	
Vitamin A	0%
Vitamin C	0%
Calcium	0%
Iron	8%

Label B

Nutrition Facts
Per 4 cookies (30g)
Servings Per Container 8

Amount	%Daily Value
Calories 130	
Fat 4g	6%
Saturated Fat 1g +Trans Fat 1g	10%
Cholesterol 0mg	
Sodium 80mg	3%
Carbohydrate 23g	7%
Fibre 0g	0%
Sugars 6g	
Protein 2g	
Vitamin A	0%
Vitamin C	0%
Calcium	0%
Iron	8%

First we read and compare the Nutrition Facts:

1. **Serving Size:** Although the weight is the same for both serving sizes (30 g), the first serving size is for 2 cookies and the second is for 4. How many cookies would you really eat? (Twenty-five is the wrong answer!)
2. **Calories**: The calories are too close to call. Remember, the amount of calories is less important than the quality of those calories. Calorie counting can become complex and confusing, so let's keep it simple. The other nutritional facts tell us what kind of calories are in the cookies. It's what makes up the calories that counts.

3. **Fat**: A contains almost double the amount of B.
4. **Saturated Fat**: A contains triple the amount of B.
5. **Sugar**: A has a bit more sugar than B.
6. **Fibre**: Pretty close; 1 g of fibre in A is negligible, and B has none.

Now that you know the facts, which cookie did you choose?

Of course, the right answer is Neither! If you were paying attention, you would remember that you should buy neither of these cookies because they both contain trans fats.

Going Nuts

This is a comparison of the nutrients in shelled tree nuts and peanuts. Use your label-reading skills to decide which ones you want to be snacking on. They are all good sources of healthy fats and protein, as well as a host of other micronutrients. Be aware of packaged (processed) nuts. Usually, they have been roasted in an unhealthy oil, are really high in salt, or perhaps roasted at too high a temperature, killing the nutrients. Buy them raw yourself and roast them in batches in the oven for 14 to 18 minutes at 350⁰ F depending on how roasted you like them (some nuts roast faster than others). Stir in some honey and add a little pink salt. Yum, on a salad these are great!

Serving Size: 1 oz. or 28 grams

Nut	Number of Nuts	Calories	Protein	Fat Total	Fat Sat	Fat Mono	Fat Poly
Almonds	20-24	160	6	14	1	9	3
Brazil nuts	6-8	190	4	19	5	7	7
Cashews	16-18	160	4	13	3	8	2
Hazelnuts	18-20	180	4	17	1.5	13	2

Macadamias	10-12	200	2	22	3	17	0.5
Peanuts	28	170	7	14	2	7	4
Pecans	18-20 halves	200	3	20	2	12	6
Pine nuts	150-157	160	7	14	2	5	6
Pistachios	45-47	160	6	13	1.5	7	4
Walnuts	7 (14 halves)	190	4	18	1.5	2.5	13

4. Eat 7 Meals a Day

Most of us eat too much at one time. Eating too much floods your body with insulin and serotonin and puts it into storage overdrive. It also leaves you feeling bloated, tired, and guilty. Another problem with overeating is that your stomach stretches and your "full" level increases. If you are habituated to keep eating until you get the full signal, then you can see how this would be problematic. This is where having your meals all ready to go for the day, will help in not overeating, by creating a structure and simple balance with your meals. With the set meal sizes and timing you will habituate your body to a new nutritional baseline.

As an example of what the meals might look like in a day I will give you what I take with me every day whether I am working or not.

> 7:30 a.m. Breakfast at home after morning wake up and before I leave: 400 g egg whites, ½ cup steel cut oats
> 9:00 a.m. Meal 1: 130 g baked chicken breast, ¾ cup of steamed cauliflower, ½ cup cooked brown rice
> 11:00 a.m. Meal 2: 130 g baked chicken breast, ¾ cup of steamed cauliflower, ½ cup cooked brown rice
> 1:00 p.m. Meal 3: 226 g baked tilapia, ¾ cup of steamed cauliflower, 100g of cooked sweet potato
> 3:00 p.m. Meal 4: 226 g baked tilapia, ¾ cup of steamed cauliflower, 100g of cooked sweet potato

Post workout shake 20 min after workout: 60 g whey isolate
7:00 p.m. Meal 5: 140 g chicken with salad, mixed veggies, and seeds
9:00 p.m. Meal 6: 140 g chicken with salad, mixed veggies, and seeds

I pack a couple of different sauces or spices to go with the meals making each one taste a little different. Things like hot sauce, no-sugar-added ketchup, tzatziki, mustard, low sodium soy sauce, and Worcestershire sauce. You can add these when cooking also for a different taste and texture altogether.

Try to remember that it takes twenty minutes for the full signal to be processed through your brain, so try to be mindful when you eat. Our bodies send hormone signals to the brain, but it takes some time for the body to register what we ate (in terms of energy and nutritional composition) and then for the correct message to be relayed. If we eat too fast, the body doesn't have time to figure out what's there; so don't eat like someone is going to take it from you.

After you eat, your blood is directed to your stomach and intestines to aid in digestion. The bigger the meal, the more blood will be directed from other body functions like the brain, leaving you drowsy. (It's not only the tryptophan in the turkey that makes you sleepy; it's also the potatoes, gravy, and everything else that you gorged on.)

Eating frequently optimizes the thermic effect of food. This is when your metabolism increases as you utilize the food you have eaten. Essentially, it's your body going to work digesting and processing your food, from chewing to processing nutrients at the cellular level. If your body is used to receiving food consistently there is no need for it to slow down and conserve energy. Everything can be running optimally. It's through this regular eating that we can rebuild our metabolism to more optimal levels, metabolism that has been struggling to find balance through years of erratic eating, starvation diets, etc.

If you like to snack, that can be okay; it's just the types of things you snack on that need to change. If you are eating every two hours, there's almost no time to snack, unless the snack is taking the place of a meal. Keep it simple. Even a snack should consist of protein and a low-glycemic-index carb. If you are hungry, eat. And remember, if you are not hungry and you are eating, raise your awareness but not your guilt as to why you are eating.

5. Plan, Prepare, and Package

Benjamin Franklin said it best: "By failing to prepare, you are preparing to fail."

Plan ahead to eat well. Even if you are away from home, you can easily prepare and bring healthy, portable snacks. Prepare your meals as if you are preparing them for your child. Not only will you be doing this soon enough, but it will make you more conscious of what you are giving yourself. If you think you don't have time to do this, you're wrong. There is no argument on this point—this is your health we're talking about. Be prepared to be carrying a bag around at all times; you will always have a meal and your water with you. When you need to start carrying a baby bag, it will be second nature. I recommend always having an extra meal or backup like a protein bar or a protein shake with you. Often things go a little longer than expected or you might get held up unexpectedly and it's always nice to know you are covered. Having peace of mind when you are starting to get hungry is vastly underrated.

Stay away from fast food joints—high fat, high sugar, high salt, high death rate. If you happen to find yourself thrown into a van, tied to a chair, held at gunpoint, and forced to eat at a fast food establishment, at least be armed with knowledge so you can make the best of the choices available. Many places serve salads (ask for a low-fat dressing) and grilled items. Ask for a whole grain (you will be lucky to get whole wheat) bun without the sauce. Beware of "home-style" items—they often have more fat and sugar than regular menu items.

6. Start Your Day Right

Eating breakfast is a critical step in your program, preparing you for the day ahead. You have been sleeping for six to eight hours, and by the time you arrive at work your body is running on fumes. Desperately seeking sugar, you will take the quickest fix, and that usually comes in the form of the foods we are trying to avoid, like candy bars, soda, or other fast-digesting carbohydrates like those infamous office donuts or the latest white flour sugar bomb *aka* a muffin at the local coffee hut.

A study at the University of Missouri examined whether a high-protein compared with a normal-protein breakfast leads to daily improvements in appetite, satiety, food motivation and reward, and evening snacking in overweight or obese, breakfast-skipping girls. The conclusions of the study were that eating breakfast led to beneficial alterations in the appetite, hormonal, and neural signals that control our food intake. Only the high-protein breakfast led to further alterations in these signals and reduced evening snacking compared with breakfast skipping, although no differences in daily energy intake were observed. These data suggest that the addition of breakfast, particularly one rich in protein, might be a useful strategy to improve satiety.

7. Leave a Little on Your Plate

Eating until you are satisfied—that is, not hungry—is an excellent way for you to optimize your body's fuel use. Another quick way to judge how much protein and carbohydrate you are getting in a meal is to use your hand, a suitable serving size of carbohydrates being the size of your fist, and protein, the size of your palm. This may seem small at first, but remember, we are retraining our bodies. Smaller-sized portions shrink our stomach, keeping our metabolism stoked and running at an optimal rate. Conversely, the portions might seem large and it may seem like all you do is eat, but you are in all probability eating this many calories already. You are just not eating real food but items that are more recognized as "snacks," like chips, muffins, granola bars, candy bars, etc. This disconnected and automatic eating when we grab a snack or open the cupboard to grab something to put in our mouths will become more apparent to you when you start to replace the junk with a solid structure containing real food. You may find yourself wanting to eat the sugary sweet or salty snack when you have just eaten and are not hungry or maybe even as you are eating your prepared meal. This provides a great opportunity to raise awareness around the fact you are wanting to feed something other than your body.

The secret is don't let yourself get too hungry or be caught without the means to feed yourself properly. Be responsible for feeding yourself—if you just ate, know that you will be doing so again in two hours.

In the first few weeks, you may feel angry, frustrated, and resentful with your new way of eating. You will probably be calling me all sorts of names and saying, "What does this Scott guy know anyway!" Don't worry, I won't take it personally. This is your body in withdrawal. Withdrawal is something our culture tends to flinch at and even considers a negative, something to try and avoid, whereas in reality, it is something to be honoured and respected. It is your body trying to heal itself, trying to regain its natural balance. What is hollering at you is that ugly little face that separated you from yourself when you fed it what it wanted; it's now panicking and trying to find a way to survive. It's craving those big calorie bombs or sugar rushes or maybe the sedation that comes from a big greasy meal.

DO NOT WORRY. YOU WILL GET OVER THIS.

Anger, cravings, and looking for someone to blame are normal and only temporary responses to withdrawal. Keeping yourself fueled will help your resolve and allow you to be more able to discern between what is fact and fiction in your head. Eating every two hours will keep you energized, help conquer cravings, and keep you safe with simple structure. Your body will adapt to your new way of eating.

It takes about two or three weeks to feel and adjust to the effects of a dietary change physically. Along with an improved sense of taste, you will soon start to be more aware whenever you try to put negative things in your body.

Eat Like a King!

- Eat six to seven smaller meals a day; eat every two (maximum three) hours.
- Eat protein and carbs at each meal.
- Stay away from juices, pop, and other processed drinks. They will fatten you up quickly.
- Drink 12 to 16 cups of water daily.
- Use quality protein drinks and bars in emergencies or when you are strapped for time. Pick ones with natural ingredients.
- Never shop when you're hungry or without a grocery list.
- Have a high calorie meal once a week. Eat the foods you have been craving, and ask yourself what the underlying feeling of the craving might be. This meal will have physiological benefits like keeping the body guessing, and psychological benefits like helping maintain a sense of perspective, increasing awareness, and providing short-term focal points. So, when things seem like they are getting tough to stay within your structure or you are tempted at work or a social event, you can say, "I can have it Saturday," to help remove the feeling of denial.

- Plan and pack your day's food and never let yourself get hungry—that's when you make unhealthy eating decisions.

If you think your relationship with food is not that complex or something you can change and manipulate as you wish, you may of course be right. I would, however, like you to think about our history with food, not as a species but as individuals. When we are born and come screaming into this world, one of the first things we are given, hopefully after some direct human contact, is food. Either a breast or a bottle is offered to us in our heightened emotional state, serving to nourish, soothe, and comfort us. We are given our sustenance by those caring for and protecting us, so food is linked with

- Safety
- Sustenance
- Survival
- Attachment
- Emotional nurturing
- Love

These fundamental and powerful human needs are attached to food and are a connection established from our first breaths. Now think about that and the depth of effect within each of us. Now think if you were going to develop a product with a highly motivated and easily manipulated market. Hmm! The food companies know this and know exactly what they are doing, which is why they produce what they do to keep us coming back for more.

Don't get me wrong. Food is not addictive, real food that is. When you eat real food, you get healthier, stronger, faster, smarter, and more emotionally balanced. Reflect on a period of your life when you ate good food. You will notice that with good things, good energy happens; with negative things, negative energy happens. This works with food, thoughts, and perspectives. Raise your awareness around this and start to make a conscious shift.

Some individuals may have the standpoint (which is common amongst the stereotypical tough guy or man's man), "I'll eat whatever the heck I want. No one's going to tell me what to eat!" This is the "Rebel." The irony behind this type of viewpoint is you are eating exactly what "they" want you to and not being a rebel at all; you are just betraying yourself. Be a true rebel and go against the norm. Don't follow the herd. Start to care about what you put into your body and what happens around you.

By doing this you will show your child how to know, care, and be strong for themselves.

Life owes me nothing, yet offers me everything.

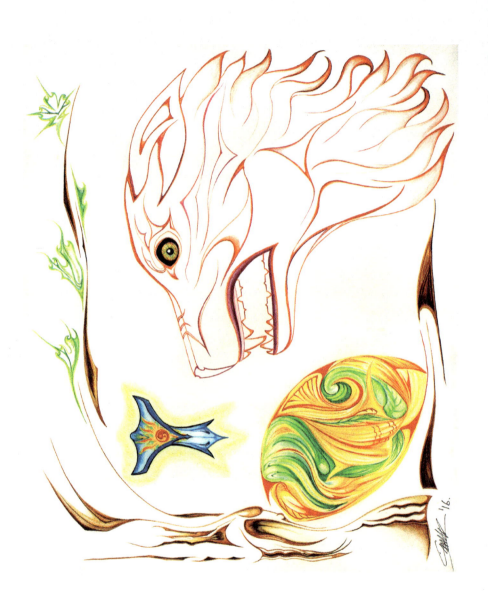

Chapter 9 The Phase 3 Workout

At the beginning of our journey, we gather our courage and strength contemplating change and then through a first step we actually begin to take action, transitioning knowledge to application, and gaining knowledge through application.

Balanced change—the kind we are working on here—most often occurs in a progressive manner. At first, the change will be overall with changes tending to come quickly. We will feel and clearly see the differences made by our efforts. Performing the workouts, increasing our self-awareness, and changing how we nourish our bodies will all still be fresh and stimulating both physically and mentally.

As we consistently implement our growth techniques and develop new behaviours, our body and mind begin to become efficient and familiar with our new ways of being. As we adapt, progress and change start to level off. It is at this point when an adjustment is required to continue growth and stimulate change (part of the reason why each phase is different).

The Principle of Increasing Contrast

We are not taught, encouraged, or accustomed to hold a perspective of balanced progressive change developed on a foundation of truth. In our society, we are taught in a very closed rigid environment. We are sold on quick fixes, with superficial win-or-lose, pass-or-fail stances, popping pills or validating excuses as to "why it didn't work." If we work out for a month and our arms are firm and our shoulders are strong but we "still don't have a six pack," it is like we failed.

This is where the "Principle of Increasing Contrast" begins to take effect.

It is also at this point where progress is still made but at a slower rate than the substantial gains experienced at the beginning of the program. The changes we see move from overall changes to more specific or focused areas. It may seem like we are working just as hard with less and less progress.

We now have parts of ourselves that have transformed; for example, firmer arms and other parts that still have a greater potential for change, such as fat around the belly. This is a dissimilarity that had not been present before, creating a type of awareness within us that was also not there before.

This is an inappropriate emphasis of negatively perceiving a positive event.

There is incongruence between the reality of what is happening and our self-perception. We are not used to seeing ourselves in positive or empowering ways. The reason for this is our application of a negative perspective may be well-practised, whereas positivity is not nearly as familiar. So as the contrast between what has changed and what has not increases, so does our unbalanced perception of them.

This may sound familiar; that's because the critic is up to its tricks again, this time trying to take advantage of the transition in your growth. The same uncertainty you felt at the beginning of the journey has returned. The critic still has a good foothold, because we are still becoming familiar learning and implementing our new ways of coping. The old ways, which support the critic and its lies and negativity, see their chance to get back in. This is new territory, which is exciting and what we have been striving for. In truth, it is a cause for celebration, though with the thrill and excitement of a new look and pending

Chapter 9

fatherhood comes uncertainty through which the whispers of the critic can be heard. It is through the new mixture of success and doubt that the critic tries some new angles of attack.

It's the old self versus the new self.

We have programmed ourselves to look for weakness so we can estimate our chances of success in a given situation. Unless the odds are stacked in our favour, our propensity is to err on the side of caution, thinking that the safe bet is to do nothing and stay status quo, never doing anything and never going anywhere.

This principle applies not only to our physical changes but also to the behavioural, emotional, and spiritual wakefulness you will be experiencing on this journey. As our self-awareness increases, we should remain cognizant that some aspects take a little longer to change than others.

Combat this just as you did in the beginning. Let go and keep it simple. Stick to the plan and trust what has worked thus far and it will continue to do so.

This is where taking a look at the picture and wish you wrote for yourself at the beginning of your journey will help bring you back to your foundation. Not only will this be a reminder to maintain the fence around the vulnerabilities of your truth and what it protects, but a recognition of how far you have come. Take a moment now to reflect on this.

I am not suggesting here that you now see yourself as wonderful and all knowing, and run down the street bare-assed screaming "I'm free, I'm free!" That would not be a congruent way to perceive yourself at the current moment. Open yourself to getting familiar with who you are, and really let go. What I am suggesting is that you start with becoming more aware of how you get in your own way.

- Identify
- Acknowledge

- Accept
- Then decide what if anything you would like to see change.

Change

One of the most difficult things for humans is change. Change is the unknown, where our wonderfully creative minds run wild fabricating scenarios and inducing fear.

What we have knowledge of are the various outcomes of our learned behaviours. Regardless of how undesirable the consequences may be, the behaviours, feelings, and outcomes are familiar (when I do this, this happens) and through that familiarity, there is security, a type of comfort, leaving us only having to justify and rationalize why we do what we do, which is easy enough when we are not truthful with ourselves.

There is no internal script, no knowledge of what will happen when you change your established behaviour to a new one. Just the thought of losing habits and coping mechanisms that have been "shielding and comforting" you will make you anxious, uncertain, and fearful, even if those coping mechanisms have a negative consequence. The known outcome is still favoured over the unknown.

Anxiety, uncertainty, and fear are powerful emotions and the irony is that as we try to change our coping, our emotions become more pronounced. With heightened emotions, our automatic response is to implement the very coping mechanisms we are trying to change (argh).

The brain knows what it wants and how to get it. It's our emotional brain that drives the subconscious decision-making processes. This is a physiological process through which hormonal responses and neuronal pathways are established with specific coping mechanisms for specific outcomes; our conscious mind has little to do with this process; the little brain in the back can run the show.

We need to reset ourselves and keep it simple. The first thing to do is become familiar with feeling again rather than reacting, denying, or avoiding. Find out who you are and not who everyone else has been saying you should be.

Something I have heard a lot over the years is the desire to move geographically, either by going on vacation, or by moving to another city, a better neighborhood, a nicer house. Well, the idea is not wrong though the journey lies within us and the distance we must travel is not measured by space but through time and the consistent application of our truth.

Imagine a cart travelling on a well-worn country road. The ruts in the road are deep and it takes a considerable amount of strength to break the cart free from the ruts. Once out, the cart may fall back in once in a while, but if the momentum is kept up, it is not as hard to break it free again. Over time as the cart travels, there is more distance put between the old ruts and the new path the cart is on. Now, it heads in a fresh direction towards an open horizon. Stay focused and present for the bumpy parts; once we get through them, they are always the most rewarding.

One thing you can do is to focus on the present and the fact you are doing something positive for your family and yourself. Change may seem slow, but it will continue to come and will make a huge difference in your life over the long term. Put yourself in the process; whatever you are doing, do your best at it. In the moment, you will allow yourself to experience and take joy in what you are doing, remembering that this is all new and uncomfortable and that is the way it's supposed to be.

These examples may not directly apply to you but you will have behaviours, thoughts, and reactions that have the same preventative, dissociative effect.

Watch out for words like "realistic, responsibility, maturity, obligation, sensible, prudent, practical" and "security"; these are some of the preferred words in our society that can be used for us to hide behind.

"I'm just being realistic. I am 35 years old. How can I have a body like a 20-year-old?"

"I have far too many responsibilities to exercise regularly."

"I am being sensible. It's not practical for me to eat every two hours."

This perspective is bought and paid for. Western societies are based on extrinsic motivators and external validation. We are heavily invested in a superficial and materialistic value system.

I am saying, learn how you apply this perspective; get to know the many forms your "reasons," "excuses," and "attitudes" come packaged in. Please remember not to learn this in a negative or self-deprecating way. You are getting to know an awesome individual. Give him a chance and start with just listening.

The Phase 3 Workout

Monday

> **Target Muscle Groups: Chest and Triceps**

20-Minute Morning Shot of Adrenaline

When: before breakfast

Reps

20 jumping jacks
10 step-ups per side
8 wide leg planks with alternating arm pull per side
Perform as many sets as you can in 20 minutes. Rest as little as possible. Push yourself to go as fast as you can while maintaining proper form. Because you want to work the muscles harder, start each exercise more slowly to allow the blood flow to the muscle to increase.

20-Minute Body Sculpting

When: anytime during the day

Reps

8 push-ups on ball or chair
8 chair dips
8 fly on ball
8 triceps push-ups
Perform 3 sets within 20 minutes, with minimal to no rest time between exercises. Rest and have some water between sets, no more than 2 minutes.

If you cannot finish 3 sets within the 20 minutes, drop the weight for each exercise. If you find it easy, do as many sets as you can within the 20-minute period.

Chapter 9

Wednesday

> **Target Muscle Groups: Back and Biceps**

20-Minute Morning Shot of Adrenaline

When: before breakfast

Reps

30 running on the spot with knees high
10 push-ups
40 squat punches
Perform as many sets as you can in 20 minutes. Rest as little as possible. Push yourself to go as fast as you can while maintaining proper form.

20-Minute Body Sculpting

When: anytime during the day

Pull with your elbow not your hand for the first three exercises and keep your elbow motionless for the fourth, moving only your forearm.

Reps

8 towel rows wide (overhand grip)
8 towel rows narrow (underhand grip)
8 dumbbell bent over rows
8 concentration curls on ball or chair
Perform 3 sets within 20 minutes, with minimal to no rest time between exercises. Rest and have some water between sets, no more than 2 minutes. If you cannot finish 3 sets within the 20 minutes, drop

the weight for each exercise. If you find it easy, do as many sets as you can within the 20-minute period.

Friday

> **Target Muscle Groups: Shoulders and Legs**

20-Minute Morning Shot of Adrenaline

When: before breakfast

Reps

15 push-ups
30 side-to-side jumps holding arms out
10 per side: snatch press alternating
Perform as many sets as you can in 20 minutes. Rest as little as possible. Push yourself to go as fast as you can while maintaining proper form. On your presses, keep your hands out so your arm forms a 90° angle.

20-Minute Body Sculpting

When: anytime during the day

Reps

8 squats with press
8 straight leg deadlifts with press
8 rear deltoid on ball
8 lunges with lateral raise
Perform 3 sets within 20 minutes, with minimal to no rest time between exercises. Rest and have some water between sets, no more than 2 minutes. If you cannot finish 3 sets within the 20 minutes, drop the weight for each exercise. If you find it easy, do as many sets as you can within the 20 minute period.

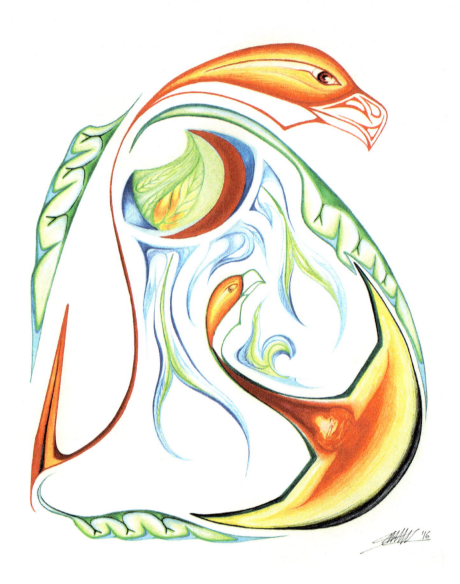

Chapter 10 Supporting Your Partner in the Third Trimester (The Home Stretch)

What She's Experiencing: 12 Common Features of the Third Trimester

1. **Feeling physically uncomfortable**: She may appreciate massages, pillows for support, and a heating pad on her lower back.
2. **Body aches and pains**: Specifically sore hips, back, feet, ankles, and ribs (not sure why I said "specifically"). All you can do is try and make it less agonizing.
3. **Feeling and being puffy**: Bloating through water retention.
4. **Sleeping difficulties**: Inability to get comfortable. She may snore.
5. **Restricted breathing**: Getting winded and tiring more easily.
6. **Lower sex drive or none at all**: Aren't you glad you listened to my advice in the second trimester?
7. **Lowered appetite**: Although she usually has little to no nausea by this point, she might have room only for small meals. But she'll have to eat more often.
8. **Impatience**: She'll be ready for the pregnancy to be over, and excited to get that baby out!
9. **Fear of labour**: As men, we will never understand the pain or fears related to labour. Whatever you do, don't start a story such as "When I was playing football and I twisted my …." Receptive support is the best we can do.

10. **Nesting urges:** Preparing for baby. Lots of shopping and planning and setting up!
11. **Fashion sense will be out the window:** I guess it's hard to see all the way around? I don't know, just use consideration and carefully chosen words if you decide to comment on her attire—remember some things can't be unsaid.
12. **Breast changes:** Her breasts will be super sensitive, possibly tender to touch, and may be leaking colostrum (a yellowish goo). This is the first type of milk produced for the baby by your partner, very rich in nutrients, antibodies, and other good stuff, to give your little one a good start. If breast feeding is not an option, don't worry there are lots of great options for you.

Ya, I know, right! So, if she is a little less patient, it's only because she is constantly uncomfortable, in pain, swollen, can't sleep, can't breathe, and is leaking. So, really it's no small miracle you haven't woken up in the middle of the night with her standing over you, frying pan in hand and a twitchy eye.

What the Average Male Is Going Through

- The 5th wheel syndrome (feeling left out)
- Weight gain (sympathy pounds)
- Excitement, anxiety, fear, and/or terror
- Sexual frustration and insecurity

Things You Can Do to Strengthen Your Relationship and Your Role in the Pregnancy

All the support and patience you have shown up to this point have been training and practice for this, the third trimester. Physically, as we have just gone over, she will be in pretty rough shape, in man terms anyway (there's a reason we don't have the babies).

This is the time your partner needs you the most physically and emotionally. You ARE the man you hoped you would be! And the man your partner and child need. Even if you have been more or less on the sidelines (or just felt that way), it's not too late to get in the game.

If you don't know what to do, start with something small: some peppermint foot massage cream, or run her a bath accompanied by candles and her favourite beverage (and join her or just sit alongside and chat). Ask if she would like you to rub some cream on her tummy. Talk to your child as you do and you will be connecting with your whole family in one beautiful moment.

Brush up on your massage techniques—it's a great way to connect and support her without being intrusive or Mr. Fixitall. Remember that all she really wants right now is just to feel normal—even a little relief would be a delight.

Bonus Tip #5

If you didn't know this already, your pregnant partner doesn't fart. Keep any opposing observations to yourself, no matter how much your eyes are watering.

Sex and the Third Term

At this point, it has been a long haul for both of you. You may be starting to feel the sting of being left out, and the passion of the second trimester is just a treasured memory.

Sex in the third trimester is definitely different. Though your doctor says the baby can't feel it, that may not be the real problem. The real problem may be that you can feel the baby! Either under your hands or against your stomach. Whatever the case may be, you feel the baby and can imagine it saying, "Get off my mom, perv!" (If you weren't going to, you probably will now. Sorry about that.)

Your partner is not comfortable doing anything in any position, never mind having sex in any position. Do not fret—this is the time you can get creative. Besides, since when did having sex and being comfortable need to go together? There are lots of ways to get the job done for both of you.

Take advantage of her hypersensitivity: get a feather.

She will be having very explicit dreams at this point, so keep this in mind and look for any signals she sends your way.

Take this as an opportunity to discuss alternatives and expand your sexual repertoire. This will have its benefits after the baby has arrived, so keep the communication going.

If you stop being intimate altogether, don't worry—it's not uncommon. As long as you are both talking about it and you're not letting the crazy train run through your head or acting like a spoiled brat, you can survive a few months. It will be all the better when the time comes to connect again.

Take Care of Yourself

This is usually the time when men start to feel a little more conflicted with what is going on and where they are personally.

You are not yet a father, yet you may be starting to feel tied down by the pregnancy. You may be trying to squeeze in all the "one last times," while around you it may look like people who are unfettered by children are making plans and moving ahead with their lives. You may be thinking of the "what ifs."

Don't feel badly about these thoughts. Some people will tell you they are natural and everyone goes through it. Well, they are and they are right. Remember what we talked about when it comes to new possibilities and positive self-perception? The same doubt and fear will be present here. Being a father is about as big a job as anyone can hold. To know that that is what you will be requires you to honour and trust

Chapter 10

yourself to even consider the task. So that is a pretty big change in self-opinion; it's a pretty big change in everything.

Well, it's the same thing here as before. Human beings tend not to like change, even positive change. These thoughts will come and go. Know that they're just your fears, your inner critic trying to stay alive. As we also already know, fear is contrived within your mind. Do not let it tarnish your gift and your ability to enjoy it. I guarantee you that as soon as you see your little angel, the joy will hit you like a lightning bolt and put all of your worries into perspective.

If it doesn't feel real for you and you feel like you're not there ("there" being where your partner and all her friends seem to be), go out by yourself and buy or even make something for your new family member. A first gift from DAD!

A wonderful way to savour the anticipation is to visit the baby nursery of the hospital, if you plan to deliver in one. Utilize this opportunity when you do your "dry run" to the hospital, to know your route, where to park, how and when to pay, the proper entrance to use, best procedures, etc. You and your partner will feel the magic in the air. Take a deep breath as you imagine your baby in your arms. My advice is to enjoy this moment and don't miss out on it. Make the time to utilize the same visualization techniques we applied in the other aspects of the program. Be aware to prepare.

Not only should you be trimming the fat on yourself, but on your lifestyle also. How do you waste your time? Yes, I said waste. Do you watch television, surf the internet, or play video games? Soon enough, it will seem like you have no time. If you cut out the crap now, you will have more time for the things that will enrich your life. What I am trying to say here is prioritize what is important. If you like playing video games, make time, but not at the expense of your self-care (workouts, grocery shopping, cooking, sleeping, spending time with your partner, etc.). Remember, if you don't take care of yourself, it will have a negative impact on your life and the lives of those you love.

The same logic applies here as to the oxygen mask principle. If you are in a plane with your family and the oxygen masks fall, what do you do? You may think, "Take care of my kids, of course, and put their masks on!" No. You need to get your mask on first. Unforeseen variables will happen and unless you are in a position to help with your wits and your strength in place, everyone is in jeopardy.

This is a great way to identify detrimental coping. If a behaviour does get in the way of supportive activities, clearly it's neither a productive nor a positive aspect of your life. This is another great opportunity to be curious and ask yourself, "What am I using this to hide from or avoid?" Remember to do it openly and gently, leaving space for the answer and not filling the silence with conjecture.

The Last Few Weeks

A spa day or a day at the salon close to her due date might be a nice surprise for your partner. She has a lot of things on her mind and time for primping is probably not high on the list. Also, she will probably appreciate it after the birth, when visitors show up and lots of photos are taken. (If you make the appointment, be sure to tell the spa that she's pregnant and how far along.)

Make sure you have the pantry full and lots of ready-to-eat frozen meals. (These will be homemade, of course, or at least whole food.)

Preparations You Can Do

- If your home doesn't already have them, install smoke alarms and CO_2 detectors.
- Make sure you have booked time off work so you can be there to help, and to soak up this wonderful time.
- Find out if your mother-in-law or other visitors are coming to stay. Work with your partner to arrange accommodation,

transportation, and any other needs your visitor might have.
- Make a list and pack your bags for the hospital. Try to think of everything each of you will need: lip balm, her favourite drink, slippers, underwear, snacks, something to read, phone numbers, phone rechargers, toiletries, and makeup. And don't dare forget the camera, with freshly charged batteries (bring extras, too), and extra memory cards.
- Keep the car gassed up and tuned up.
- If it's winter and you live where there might be snow, make sure you have good snow tires on.
- Buy or make a gift for your partner to give to her on the day of the birth, to show her how much you love her and appreciate all she has been through.
- Print out a checklist and put it on the fridge; put another copy in the "birth bag."

Labour

Your partner knows her body best, so if she says she's in labour, take it as what's happening. You don't want to be the reason she gave birth on the side of the road. Even if what's called "false labour" happens a couple of times, your support is what she needs. False labour is also called Braxton Hicks contractions; they are the body getting ready for the real thing. Ask your doctor about them if they are a concern for you. Taking a walk or giving her a massage is something that will help with these. A massage, warm shower, or towels on her back will also be something to do when she is in actual labour. Be sure to ask her if it's helping and have a few different options.

If your partner has false labour and you rush to the hospital in the middle of the night, she will feel awkward enough, so keep any negative comments or stating the obvious to yourself. Look at it as a practice run: How did you handle it? Did you forget anything?

We are not going to get into the particulars of delivering a baby here. Those are facets of this journey that you should discover on your own. You can do that by going to a pre-natal class with your partner (which I highly recommend). It's a great way to put time aside (scheduled) just for the two of you specifically around the pregnancy. Make it a special part of your week and go out for a meal either on the way there or on the way home. Another good option is discussing the upcoming event and what to expect with your midwife or doctor.

There is lots going on and emotions are about as high as they can get. Unexpected things happen. There are lots of bodily fluids during the labour process. Often there is a fair amount of blood during the delivery. If you are in the hospital, the medical team will take care of clean up and are trained for possible variables. Don't forget, you still have a say, though you definitely do not want to get in the way. You are still going to be the person that has to live with either your action or inaction.

While my youngest son was being delivered, our doctor was itching his face on my wife's leg. She looked at me and I was unsure of what to do. The female obstetrician was the one in charge and our doctor was just hanging out on my wife's leg. Why am I telling you this? Well, I feel I should have said something either to him or to my wife. If I had been practising the methods laid out in this book, I would have been more sure of who I was and been able to speak or not speak from my truth. My uncertainty came with the mistrust I had in myself.

Now the one exception to speaking your truth during this event is with your partner. She will be very possibly running the full gamut of emotions: happy, scared, sad, in pain, euphoric, frustrated, exhausted, etc. "Yes, sweetheart" and "No, sweetheart" are your options. Make a judgment call—maybe not even that—that whatever she is feeling or saying is correct (and "perfectly sane"). Do not, for the sweet love of puppies, try to correct her!

Epilogue

Congratulations! You have made huge strides in increasing your awareness. Through this you will have the ability to see and understand what your priorities truly are. You will be able to seize opportunities to learn and become stronger rather than default into a guilt/shame spiral. So when or if you miss a day or two or more of your exercises or putting your meals together, see it for the opportunity that it is to gain more awareness of that negative voice. Don't forget to celebrate the fact that you are even aware of the change in your structure.

It's pretty cool when you think about it. You have "problems" in *areas* where you never had areas before. Remember it's a process and just like consistent curls build a bicep, consistent honesty builds awareness. Both are also similar in that if you stop applying that which stimulates them, they will begin to atrophy.

This is wonderful awareness to have going into your beautiful journey. Your life will be full of new and unfamiliar experiences and dealing with the negative voice is a challenge even at the top of our game. When you are sleep-deprived and changing a diaper in the middle of the night with a beautiful little voice screaming at the top of its lungs, that will be the time to apply your truth and the awareness you have learned through this book. This will allow you to have gratitude and to see your gift.

Find success in life by meeting failure everyday.

Appendix A Exercise Details

Ball Punch Crunches

- Lie on your back with the ball under your mid to lower back. The closer it is to your hips, the greater the resistance.
- You may feel compelled to lift your head, putting unnecessary stress on your neck muscles. Keep your head neutral in Foundational Form.
- Hold your hands either by your cheeks or at your shoulders (whichever is more comfortable as long as you keep your shoulders back).
- Alternate hands in a light fist punch across your body as you come up, punching towards your hips.
- You only need to move a little to engage your abdominals.
- Hold the position at the top for a moment and use your abdominals to lower back down.
- Don't curl your back—keep it straight.

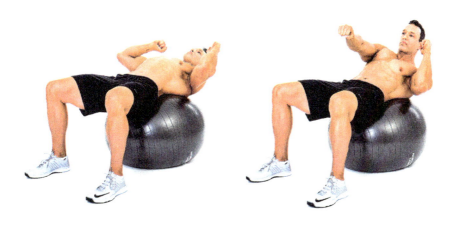

Biceps Curl

- Standing in Foundational Form bring your arm slightly forward so you can turn your hand palm up.
- Keep your upper arm motionless as though your elbow is nailed to your side.
- Bend at the elbow moving your forearm as far as you can towards your shoulder.
- Keeping resistance on the biceps muscle control arm back to start.

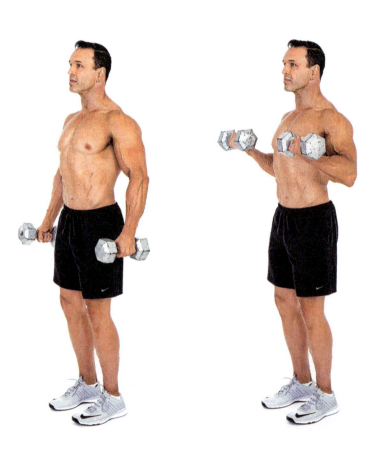

Appendix A

Bike Abs

- Lie on your back on the floor. Bend both knees and bring them up to your chest.
- Place your hands by your ears with elbows facing forward.
- Extend your right leg fully, keeping your left knee bent.
- Twist as you bring your right elbow to your left knee.
- Repeat with other leg and elbow.

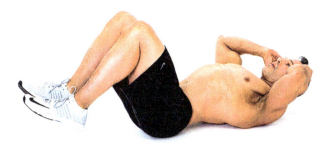

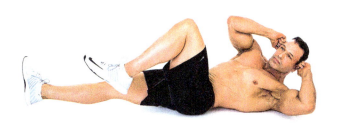

Body Wake-Up

- Stand with your arms extended in front of you. Squat until your thighs are parallel to the floor, then raise back up to standing position. If you are a little tight at the start either go as far as you can maintaining form or widen your stance.
- With your legs straight touch your quads, knees, shins, or toes, whichever your start point may be. (Do not curl your back).
- Keeping your legs straight, come back up to standing position.
- Keeping your arms straight, lift them above your head and then back down to your hips.

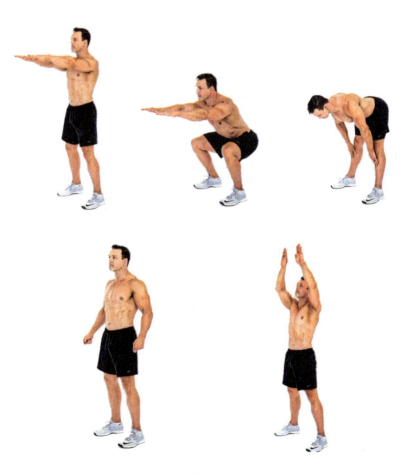

Chair Dips

- Push two chairs together just wider than shoulder width.
- Put your hands on the chairs so your arms are straight (not locked). Your arms will be at about 80° with the ground. Keep your shoulders back and chest up. Adjust your feet underneath you to lessen resistance.
- Lower yourself so that your chest is at the same level as your hands. Think about your chest working and pushing with your elbows not your hands.
- Push yourself back up. Squeeze your upper arms together with your chest muscles at the top of the movement, keeping your chest up and your shoulders back.

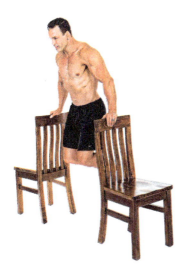
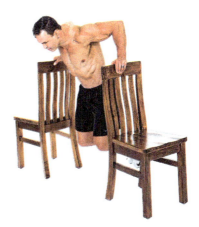

Chest Press on Ball or Floor

- Lie face up on the ball or floor with your body in Foundational Form.
- Hold your arms out to your sides (not at a 90° angle with your body but just below shoulder height) with your hands up above your elbow.
- Keeping your chest up, bring your upper arms across your chest (think about pushing with your elbows).
- Squeeze at maximal contraction and then control your arms back down to start position.

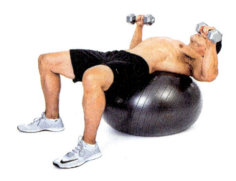

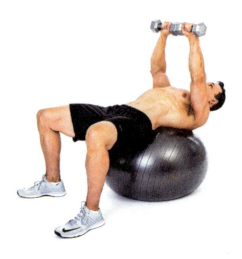

Concentration Curls on Ball or Chair

- Sitting on the ball with your feet apart and the weight between your legs, pick up the weight with your right arm.
- Keeping your shoulders square, bend forward at the hips until your upper right arm is against your inner right thigh.
- Your arm should be fully extended with the weight off the floor.
- Moving only your forearm, curl the weight up to your shoulder. Twist your hand at the top of the movement (twisting your pinky towards your face) to get maximum concentration on the biceps.
- Repeat with other arm.

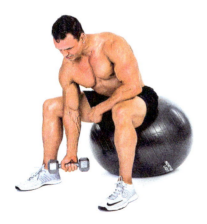
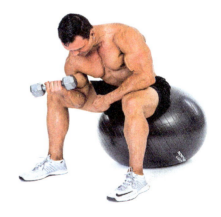

Dumbbell Bent over Row

- Stand in Foundational Form with weights in your hands, palms facing your body.
- Hinging at your hips, bend forward, letting your arms hang freely and keeping your shoulders back and your knees bent.
- With your head in a neutral position, pull your elbows towards your waist, squeezing with your back muscles (concentrate on your back, not on your biceps).
- Control the weight back down, keeping your shoulder blades back and down so you can feel the stretch through your back muscles.
- Keep the rest of your body motionless. Think of your hands as hooks and pull with the upper arm only.

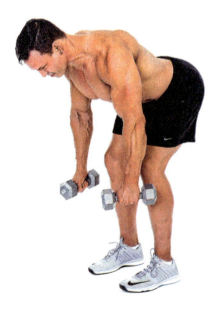
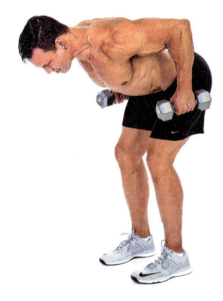

Dumbbell Military Press Seated on Ball or Chair

- Sit at the edge of the ball or chair.
- Keep your body in Foundational Form, maintaining the curve in your lower back and keeping shoulders back and down (keep your trapezoid muscles relaxed).
- Feet can be apart or together; if you are on a ball, having your feet apart will make stabilization easier.
- Keep your feet out away from you, either under your knees or further. Do not pull them back towards you.
- From shoulder level, press both arms maximally over your head keeping your shoulders down.
- Control your arms back down to your shoulders.

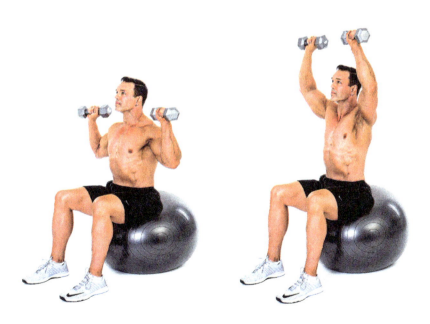

Fast Feet

- Start by standing with your left foot on the ground, right knee bent, and your right foot placed on the step or bench in front of you.
- Take your right foot off the step. As you do so, jump with your left foot, bringing it up onto the step.
- Continue alternating your feet slowly at first to develop balance and rhythm. As you become comfortable, increase your speed. Be aware in this exercise you will have an even greater tendency to curl your shoulders forward, especially when starting to get tired.
- Think about driving your knees up and pumping your arms front to back rather than across your body.
- Keep your chest up and your shoulders back and down.

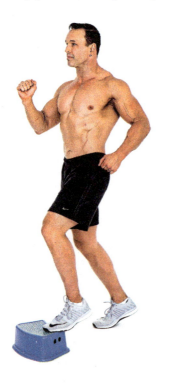
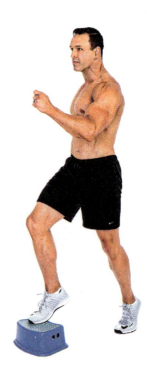

Fly on Ball or Floor

- Lie face up on the ball or floor with your body in Foundational Form.
- Hold your arms out to your sides but not straight out; at approximately an 80° angle (slightly below shoulder height), arms slightly bent.
- Keeping your chest up, bring your upper arms across your chest (think about pushing with your elbows). Squeeze at maximal contraction and then control the weight back down to starting position.

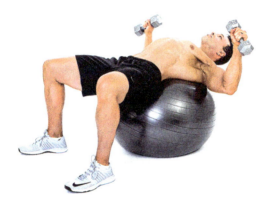

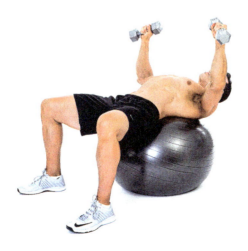

Forearm Extension on the Ball on Knees

- Start by kneeling in front of the ball with your back straight.
- Bending at the hips, place your elbows on the ball.
- Squeezing your stomach, roll forward on the ball until your body is straight from your shoulders to your feet.
- Return to start position.

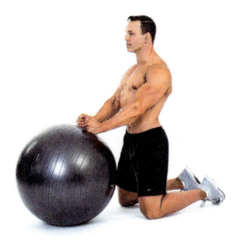

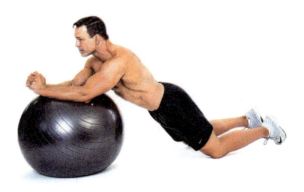

Appendix A

Guarding Stance with Leg Switch

- Fist your hands in front of your face. Leading with one hand and shoulder (facing sideways) and one leg in front of the other.
- On the same spot, jump slightly and twist your hips, switching your front leg with your back leg.
- Immediately after switching your feet, twist your upper body so you are now leading with the opposite hand and shoulder.

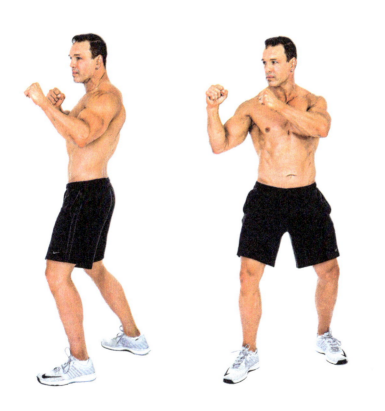

Incline Chest Press on Ball

- Lie face up on the ball or floor with your body in Foundational Form.
- Hold your arms out to your sides (not in line with your shoulders but slightly below), with your hands up above your elbow.
- With the ball just under mid to upper back, bend your knees and hinge at your hips, dropping the lower body so you are at an angle with your head higher.
- Keeping your chest up, bring your upper arms across your chest (think of pushing with your elbows). Squeeze at maximal contraction and then control your arms back down to starting position.
- This exercise is working your upper chest.

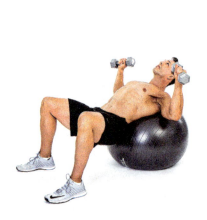
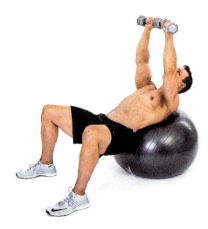

Appendix A

Jump Squats

- Perform a squat and from the bottom of the movement jump up driving with your feet and through your toes with velocity.
- As your body comes back down, begin to land with your toes gradually absorbing the landing through your feet and finally bending your knees as much as you need to minimize the impact.
- This is a power up exercise with a controlled descent.

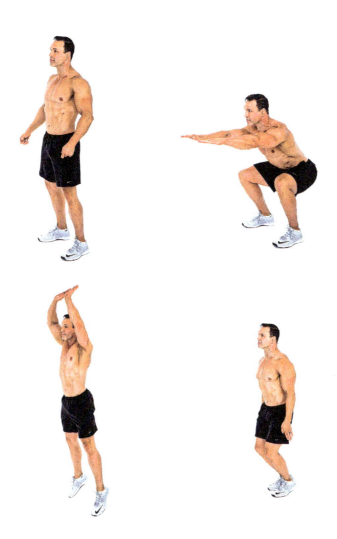

Jumping Jacks

- Perform jumping jacks starting with straight arms down at your sides and feet together.
- Raise your arms, swinging them above your head so that your hands touch. At the same time, jump your legs apart, landing on your toes with your knees slightly bent.
- End by bringing your arms back down to your sides and bringing your feet back together.

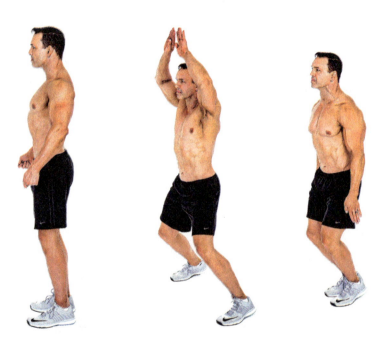

Appendix A

Lunges with Lateral Raise with or without Weights

- Stand with your feet shoulders' width apart, hands at your sides, palms in.
- Step your right leg directly forward at a 30° angle (approximate).
- Bend your right knee and lower yourself down. Make sure your knee does not go past your toes (so move downward not forward).
- As you lower your body, raise your arms at your sides leading with the elbow not the hand.
- Bend your left knee (to allow your body to continue downward) until it almost touches the ground.
- Pausing at the bottom of the movement, hold your arms as high as you can with palms facing down.
- Push through your foot with your right leg using your glutes and quads (bum and thighs) to the starting position. Lower your arms back down to your sides as you go up.

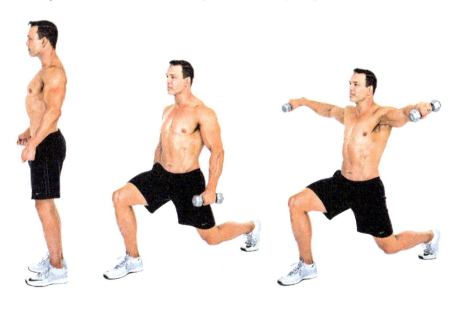

Lunges with or without Weights

- Stand with your feet shoulders' width apart, hands on your hips, and shoulders back.
- Step your right leg directly forward at a 30° angle (approximate).
- Bend your right knee and lower yourself down. Make sure your knee does not go past your toes (so move downward not forward).
- Bend your left knee (to allow your body to continue downward) until it almost touches the ground.
- Push back with your right leg to the starting position.

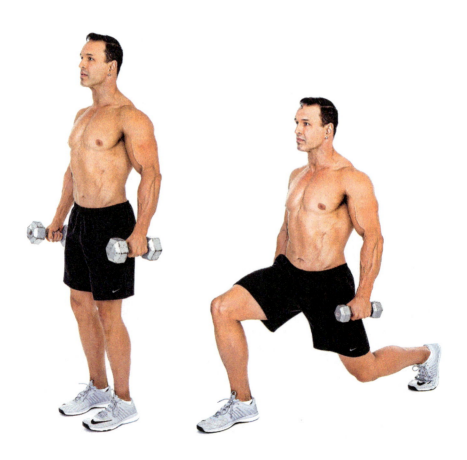

One-Arm Ball Rows

- Place your right hand and right knee on the ball, holding a dumbbell in your left hand.
- Keeping your body in Foundational Formation, hinge at the hip not the waist. Let your left arm hang with your shoulders staying back and chest up, feeling the stretch in your latissimus dorsi (the big muscle of your back).
- Pull with your elbow straight up as far as it will go, squeezing at the top of the movement then controlling it back down.
- Reverse for opposite side.

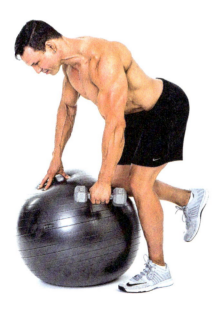
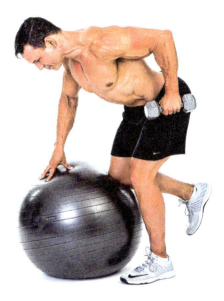

Push Pull Push-Ups

- Get into the push-up position with each hand resting on a dumbbell.
- Lower your body, maintain your body in Foundational Form.
- Push back up. At the top of the movement, pull one dumbbell off the floor as far as you can, keeping tension in your abs and glutes. With the supporting arm, hold your body as square to the floor as you can.
- Be careful not to twist too much. Pull with your elbow, squeeze your back and control the weight back down.

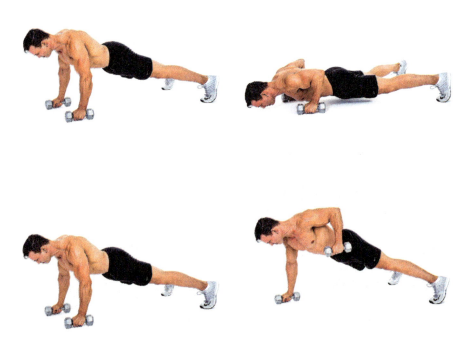

Appendix A

Push-Ups

- Get into the push-up position: hands shoulders' width apart, body in Foundational Form.
- Keeping your shoulders back and your abs tight, lower yourself to a couple of inches off the floor.
- Push back to start position.

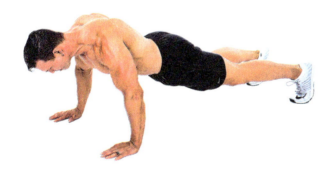

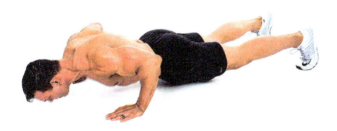

Push-Ups on Ball or Chair

- Start on your knees with your hands shoulders' width apart on the ball or chair.
- Raise your body up so you are holding it in Foundational Form.
- Perform a push-up.
- If you cannot perform the amount of reps with proper Foundational Form, try putting your knees on the ground or decreasing the repetitions.

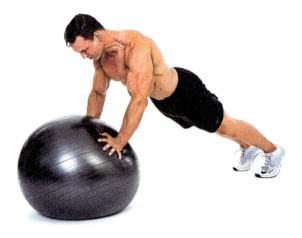

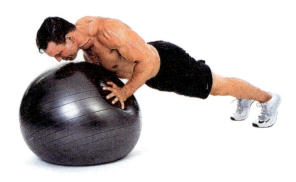

Push-Ups to Plank

- Start in the push-up position.
- Move your weight from your right hand to your right elbow and then from your left hand to your left elbow. You are now in the plank position.
- Flex your bum and abdominal muscles.
- Holding your body in Foundational Form, return to the starting push-up position, going from your elbows to your hands.

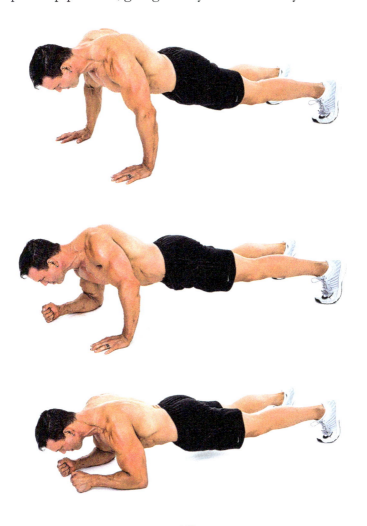

Rear Deltoid on Ball or Chair

- Sit on a bench or a ball in Foundational Form.
- Keep your torso motionless for this rear-deltoid-on-ball exercise.
- Bend forward from your hips (not waist) as far as you can while maintaining Foundational Form.
- Let your arms hang with gravity and engage the back of your shoulders, lifting your elbows up and straight out (perpendicular) to the sides of your body.
- Hold for a split second at the top of the movement, lifting your elbows as high as you can while maintaining form.
- Use the rear deltoid muscles to lower your arms to the starting position.

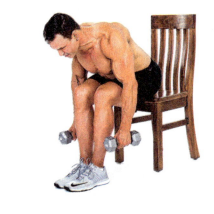

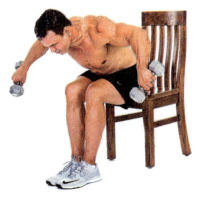

Reverse Grip Biceps Curl

- Standing in Foundational Form, bring your arm slightly forward so you can turn your hand palm down.
- Keep your upper arm motionless as though your elbow is nailed to your side. Bend at the elbow moving your forearm as far as you can towards your shoulder.
- Keeping the biceps muscle contracted, control arm back to start, keeping your palms down through the entire movement.

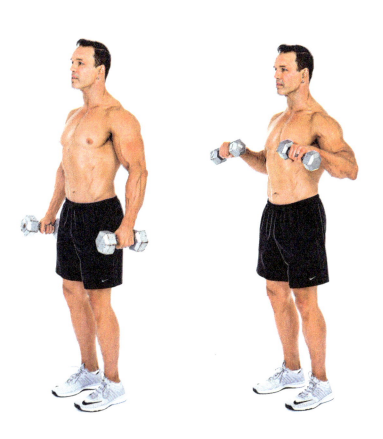

Running on the Spot with Knees High

- Stand with head and chest up shoulders back in Foundational Form.
- Move your arms front to back like you are hammering a nail.
- On the spot, drive your knees up as high as you can. Use your waist as a guide to set a level for each time you drive up your knee.
- Keep your shoulders back and maintain the curve in your lower back. As you tire, let your knees drop in height. Do not let your form diminish.

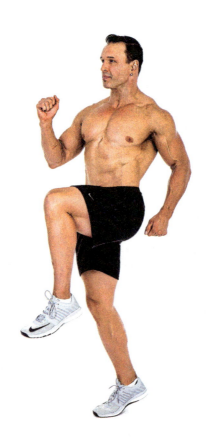

Side-to-Side Jumps

- Jump side to side on your toes keeping your feet together and your knees bent.
- Spring off your toes and land on your toes.
- Extend your arms out from your sides and hold them at shoulder height.

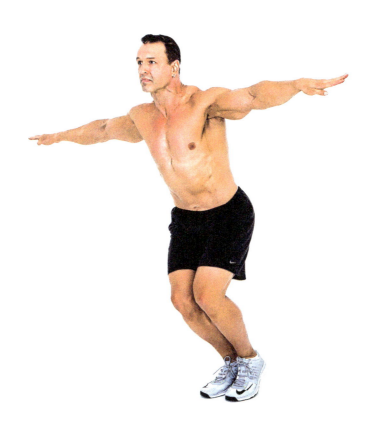

Snatch Press with or without Weights

- With a dumbbell in one hand, stand with feet shoulders' width apart and your body in Foundational Form.
- Bending at the hips and knees, let the weight hang down between your legs till it comes just below your knees.
- In a driving/jumping motion, explode upward. As you do so, pull the dumbbell to mid-chest, keeping it close to your body.
- Tuck your elbow under the weight at this point, continuing the motion using your arm and shoulder until the dumbbell is overhead.
- Alternate sides.

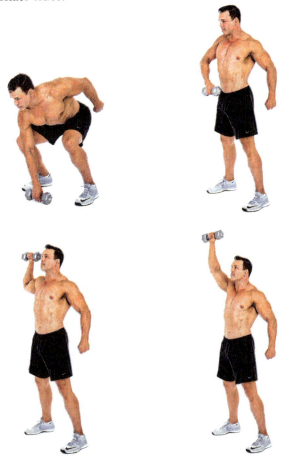

Squat

- Stand with your feet shoulders' width apart, back straight, shoulders back, and chest up. If you're using weights, have them at your sides.
- Bending your knees and your hips, squat down. Your arms may move forward, rotating at the shoulder as counterbalance (keep your shoulders back). Squat as low as you can while retaining control and Foundational Form.
- Push the floor away from you, keeping the force through your heels and the outside of your feet. Do not let your knees fold in toward each other.
- Push back to start position. Be careful not to lock your knees; keep them slightly bent. This will keep resistance on the right muscles and reduce stress on the knee joint.

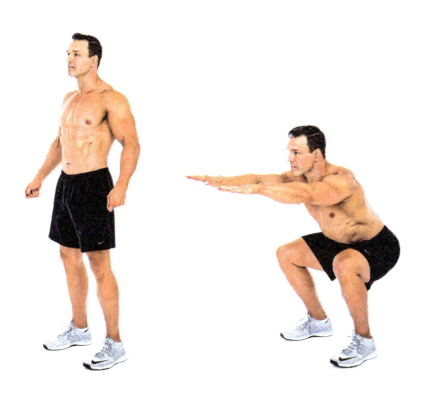

Squat Punches

- Beginning in Foundational Form, bend your knees, squatting down until you feel your quads engaging.
- Place both hands at waist level at the sides of your body in a fist, palms facing up.
- In a punching motion, extend one arm out in front of you to the mid-chest level, rotating your hand in the process, so that once your arm is extended, your palm is facing down.
- Make sure you replace your hand at the **side** of your waist palm up. Your hands will have a tendency to sneak around to the front.
- Bring that hand back and at the same time bring your other hand off your waist and forward, exchanging positions. Your fists should be passing each other at the midpoint.
- Start slowly until you become familiar with the movement. As you become more familiar and stronger, the squat can be maintained at a deeper position.

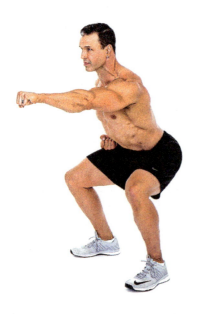
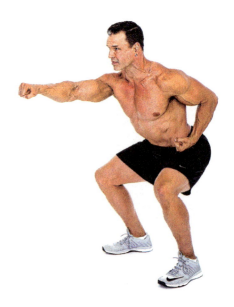

Squats with Curl with or without Weights

- Stand with your feet shoulders' width apart, back straight, shoulders back, and chest up. If you're using weights, have them at your sides.
- Bending your knees, squat down, Your arms may move forward with the weights as counterbalance (keep your shoulders back). Squat as low as you can while retaining control and Foundational Form.
- Push the floor away from you, keeping the force through your heels and the outside of your feet. Do not let your knees fold in toward each other.
- Push back to start position. Be careful not to lock your knees; keep them slightly bent. This will keep resistance on the right muscles and reduce stress on the knee joint.
- Perform a biceps curl keeping your upper arm motionless (as though your elbow is attached to the side of your body).

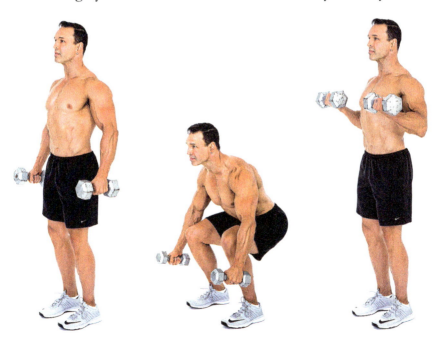

Squats with Press and No Weights

- Start these exercises easily in Phase 1 using no weights.
- Standing in Foundational Form, bend at the knees and hips as low as you can while maintaining your form, shoulders back, chest up, and lower back arched.
- From this position, driving through your heels and the outside of the feet, push yourself back up. At the top of the movement, curl your arms to shoulder height, then press your hands to maximum extension over your head, squeezing your shoulders (keep your shoulder blades back and down to prevent shrugging your shoulders).
- Do not lock your knees.

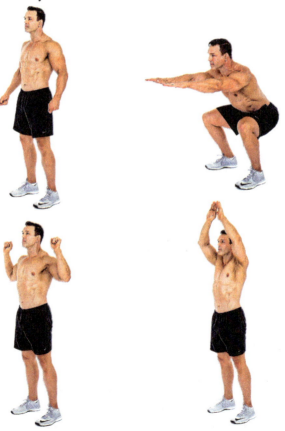

Appendix A

Squats with Press and Weights

- In Phase 2, add suitable weights.
- Standing in Foundational Form, bend at the knees and hips as low as you can while maintaining your form, shoulders back, chest up, and lower back arched. The weights should be at your side, palms facing in.
- From this position, driving through your heels and the outside of the feet, push yourself back up. At the top of the movement, curl the weight to shoulder height, then press to maximum extension over your head, squeezing your shoulders (keep your shoulder blades back and down to prevent shrugging your shoulders).
- Control the weight back down to your shoulders then to your sides.
- Do not lock your knees.

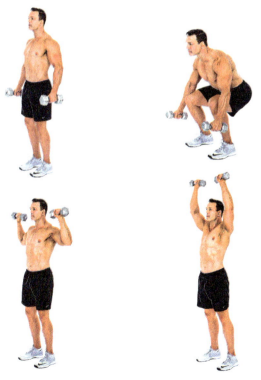

Standing Front Shoulder Raises

- Standing in Foundational Form bring your arms from your sides straight up in front of you.
- Bring them up and in to the midline of your face (both hands should be in line with both sides of your nose).
- Palms facing down.
- Lower hands back to your sides for one rep.

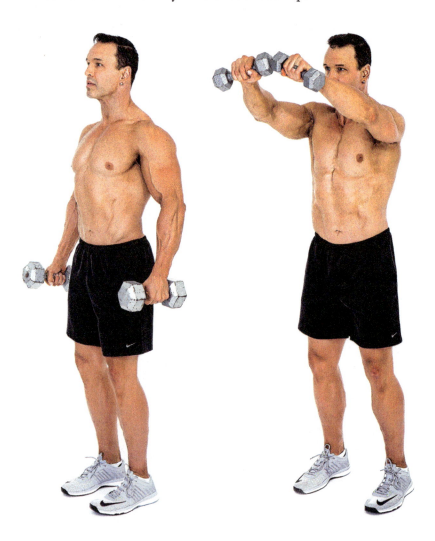

Appendix A

Step-Ups

- Stand in front of a chair, bench, or step with back straight and head up.
- Place your right foot on the chair and push, lifting yourself up until you have straightened your right leg.
- Lower yourself back to the floor replacing your right foot on the step with the left foot. Push, lifting yourself up until you have straightened your left leg.
- Lower yourself back to the floor. This is one rep.
- Repeat until rep completion or muscle fatigue.
- "With exaggerated arm movement" means to move your arms as though you were running. The counterforce is great for your core and will help you get up. This arm movement will bring your hand up in front of your face and drive your elbow back with each step.

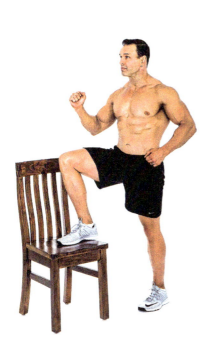
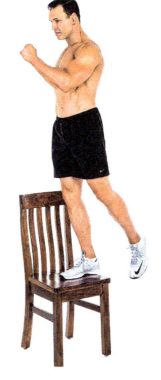

Straight Leg Deadlift

- A review of Foundational Form is recommended before starting this exercise.
- Keeping your shoulders back and maintaining the curve in your lower back are crucial elements of this exercise.
- Bend or hinge at the hips; it will feel like you are pushing your bum back. Your arms should be relaxed and hanging freely (shoulders back).
- Go as low as you can while maintaining Foundational Form. It will not be as far as you anticipated; that is a good sign you are doing it correctly.
- Pull with your hamstrings (muscles at the back of your thighs) and squeeze your glutes ("glutes" is short for gluteus maximus or bum muscle). Push your hips forward, bringing your body back to standing position.

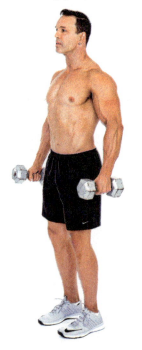
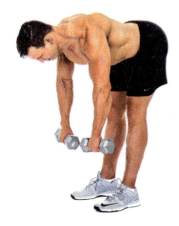

Appendix A

Straight Leg Deadlift with Press

- A review of Foundational Form is recommended before starting this exercise.
- Keeping your shoulders back and maintaining the curve in your lower back are crucial elements of this exercise.
- Bend or hinge at the hips; it will feel like you are pushing your bum back. Your arms should be relaxed and hanging freely (shoulders back).
- Go as low as you can while maintaining Foundational Form. It will not be as far as you anticipated; that is a good sign you are doing it correctly.
- Pull with your hamstrings (muscles at the back of your thighs) and squeeze your glutes ("glutes" is short for gluteus maximus or bum muscle). Push your hips forward, bringing your body back to standing position.
- Curl the weights up to shoulder height, then press fully above your head and squeeze then controlling the weight.
- Bring them back down to the shoulders and then to the waist. This is one rep.

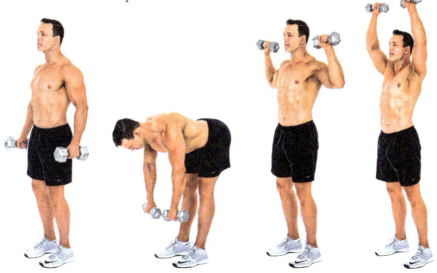

Towel Row

- Wrap a towel (you can use a sheet or a rope or anything you can hang onto) around the door handles on both sides of an open door (a tree or a pole will also do).
- Grab the towel with both hands in Foundational Form. With your feet at shoulders' width apart at either side facing the door, bend your knees, keeping your shoulders back. Adjust your feet underneath you to lessen resistance.
- As you bend your knees, lean back feeling the stretch on your back muscles.
- Pull yourself towards the door keeping your elbows close to your body squeezing your elbows back at maximum contraction. Control your body back down.
- You can adjust the intensity of the resistance by moving your feet further towards the door and away from your upper body (leaning back while holding onto the towel).

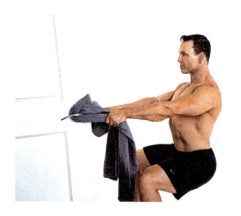
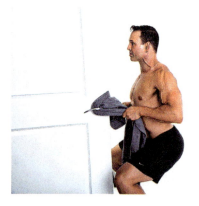

Towel Rows Narrow (underhand grip)

- Use the same posture and technique as the regular towel row, but change your hand and arm position.

- Using an underhand grip on the towel (palms facing up), keep your elbows tight to your body. This will emphasize the mid-back.

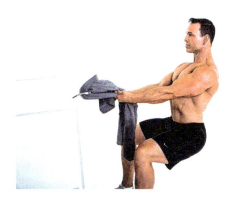
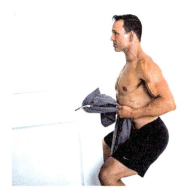

Towel Rows Wide (overhand grip)

- Use the same posture and technique as the regular towel row, but change your hand and arm position.
- Using an overhand grip on the towel (palms facing the floor), move your elbows out away from your body. This will emphasize the upper back.

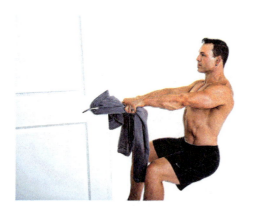 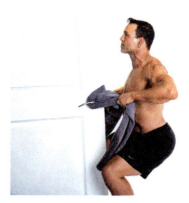

Triceps Extension on Ball or Floor

- Lie face up on the ball or floor with your body in Foundational Form.
- Hold your arms at shoulders' width apart straight out so your hands are above your head.
- Keep your elbows locked in position (do not move your upper arm). Let your forearm bend down toward the top of your head using your triceps to lower.
- Keeping resistance on the triceps throughout the movement, push your forearm back to straight arm position. Your arm should still be on an angle so gravity is still providing resistance for the triceps.

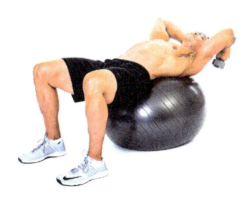

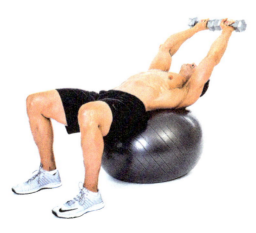

Triceps Push-up

- Get into the push-up position: hands inside shoulder-width at chest level.
- Have your fingers facing slightly out so that your palms are towards your midline.
- Maintain your body in Foundational Form.
- Keep your shoulders back and your elbows close to your body; do not let them flare out.
- Lower yourself to a couple of inches off the floor.
- Push back to starting position.

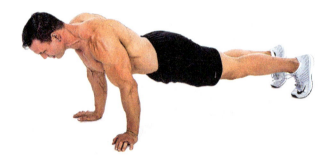

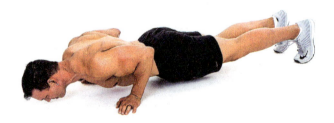

Wide Leg Plank with Alternating Arm Pull with or without Weight

- Get into the plank position with each hand shoulders' width apart resting on a dumbbell and your feet wider than shoulder width.
- Keep your body as square to the floor as you possibly can, pull the weight with one arm at a time fully contracting the latissimus dorsi (back muscle)
- Hold at the top of the movement for a count and control the weight back down.
- Repeat with the other arm.

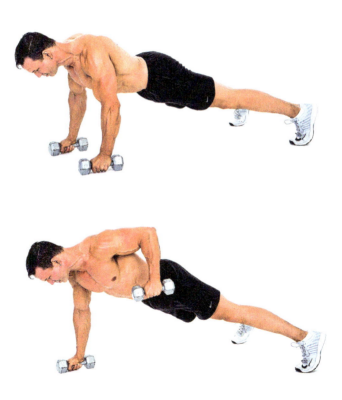

Pain is my gauge, fear is my guide.

Appendix B Stretch Details

Back (upper)

- Standing in front of a solid object, grab onto it with your left hand, bending your knees and turning in so that your left hand is in front of your right shoulder.
- Return to starting position.
- Repeat with other arm.

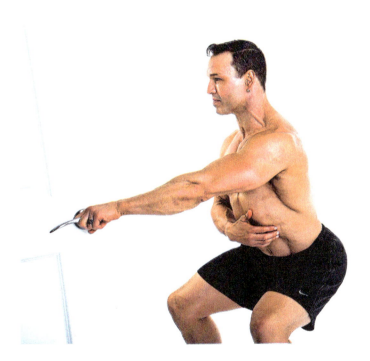

Glutes and Back

- Sitting with your back straight, put your right leg straight out and your left foot across it so your left foot is on the outside of your right knee.
- Put your right arm over your left knee and pull it towards your right.
- Repeat on other side.

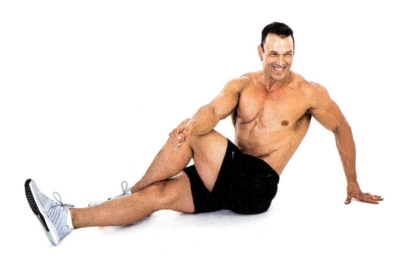

Hamstring

- Sitting with your legs apart in a V keeping your back straight and leading with your chest, reach down one leg at a time.
- Repeat on other side.

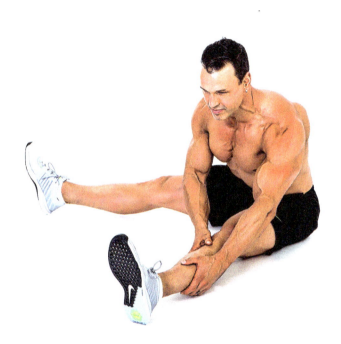

Quads

- Standing with your back to a chair, lift your left leg behind you, and put the toes of your left foot on the chair with your knee pointing down.
- Standing straight, slowly bend the right knee, dropping the body lower. Hold for 10 seconds and return to starting position.
- Repeat on other side.

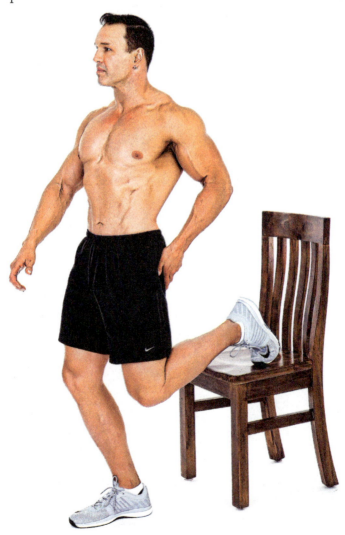

Triceps

- Take one hand and reach behind your head and grab the base of your skull. Push back with your head keeping your elbow pointing straight up. Then switch hands.
- You can increase the stretch by pushing with your head or other hand.
- Repeat on other side.

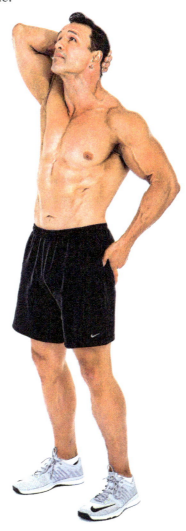

Opportunities are given.
Problems are created.

Author Biography

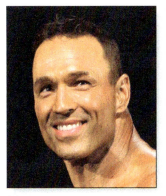

Scott Macdonald began life as a man's man, a bouncer for twenty years, a varsity football player, a biker and brawler, and a 320 lb. enforcer who didn't like many people, especially himself. He also worked in the commercial graphics industry with a self-imposed misguided work ethic where there was lots of opportunity to create inappropriate priorities which he pursued, like money, cars, motorcycles, etc. This worked well with the noise and distraction of society and the media. Even the mention of anything slightly authentic like whole food, yoga, "loving yourself," or expressing a feeling would elicit a defensive outburst or a harsh comment. His diet was beer, fast food, and keeping distracted. This negativity dragged him downward until eventually he was homeless and in and out of jail.

Today, he is a very different person:

- Husband, Father, and Grandfather
- Registered Canadian Art Therapist
- Black Belt in Taekwondo
- Professional Natural Bodybuilder
- Professional Trainer (BHK)

The cool thing about these achievements is he earned and attained them through following the principles laid out in this book.

About Scott

"THERE ARE NO PROBLEMS—ONLY OPPORTUNITIES"

Scott Macdonald
Scott specializes in supporting individuals and groups in identifying barriers to growth. Drawing upon extensive personal and professional experience, Scott illustrates the conflict we create from the resulting contradiction of our internal wisdom and externalized justification.

Currently supporting:
The Vancouver School Board
Vancouver Coastal Health Authority
The Dr. Peter Centre

Services:
If you are interested in finding your strength and exploring your truth, Scott works with all ages offering holistic support and first steps utilizing:
- Art Therapy
- Nutritional counseling
- Physical wellness
- Goal setting and assessment

Website:
www.fitforfatherhood.com

Social Media:

- Facebook: Fit for Fatherhood
- Twitter: fit4_fatherhood

CPSIA information can be obtained
at www.ICGtesting.com
Printed in the USA
LVOW05s1610210917
549562LV00037B/1169/P

9 780995 883000